RICHARD HITTLEMAN'S 30 DAY YOGA MEDITATION PLAN

RICHARD HITTLEMAN'S 30 DAY YOGA MEDITATION PLAN

RICHARD HITTLEMAN

BANTAM BOOKS · TORONTO · NEW YORK · LONDON

For Helene, Rebecca,
and the
Yoga students at Pajaro Dunes

RICHARD HITTLEMAN'S
30 DAY YOGA MEDITATION PLAN

A Bantam Book / March 1978

Photography: Thomas Burke
Illustrations: Robert Carlon
Meditators: Jeanne Muir (Secondary school teacher)
Dr. Ronald Barazani (Psychologist)
Julie Levitt (Homemaker)

ISBN 0-553-01069-7

Published simultaneously in the United States and Canada

Bantam Books are published by Bantam Books, Inc.
Its trademark, consisting of the words "Bantam Books"
and the portrayal of a bantam, is registered in the
United States Patent Office and in other countries.
Marca Registrada. Bantam Books, Inc.,
666 Fifth Avenue, New York, New York 10019.

PRINTED IN THE UNITED STATES OF AMERICA

0 9 8 7 6 5 4 3 2 1

Contents

Introduction

There is no endeavor in this life more meaningful, or of greater urgency, than the practice of meditation. It is only through quieting the mind and senses, and learning to direct the consciousness *inward*, that Self, one's true nature, can be experienced. In this experience (designated Yoga, Self-realization, *samadhi, nirvana,* the kingdom of heaven, enlightenment, God-consciousness, Universal Mind, unconditioned awareness as well as other expressions that attempt to describe the state of mergence with the Absolute), peace, knowledge, and bliss become realities. As long as one remains ignorant of Self, of who he/she really IS, suffering, anxiety, frustration, despair, restlessness, and insecurity must prevail; *without Self-recognition, there can be no fulfillment.*

Self is eternal and unchanging; It transcends duality and is without qualities (although all qualities and all things are inherent in It). Inasmuch as Self is one's true nature, the only Reality, It cannot be attained or acquired from an imagined external source. But in the way that the mind and senses usually function—captured and enslaved by the quest for gratification in an illusory, external world—Self is obscured and temporarily forgotten.

The ego, the "I," is obsessed with action. It convinces us that through its actions we will be fulfilled in the external dimension that it has constructed and maintains. So persuasive are the ego's promises that we are beguiled into identifying with its innumerable activities and, forgetting our true identity, become caught up in its relentless pursuit of fulfillment. The deeper our amnesia or hypnosis—identification

with the body, mind, senses, and their activities—the greater the obscuration of Self.

What is required, then, is the removal or dissolution of the obscuring elements, so that Self may reemerge. It is in the process of *quieting the mind* that we begin to recognize the hypnotic effect of activity and reawaken to our Reality. Once the mind and senses are stilled, the consciousness can be redirected: instead of continually flowing outward in its preoccupation with external fulfillment, it is made to journey inward to merge (effect Yoga) with its source. The application of those techniques which enable us to turn the consciousness inward and reestablish our identity as Self is the practice of meditation.

One of my books deals in detail with the Yoga and Vedanta philosophies briefly outlined above.* The subject matter of this book is devoted primarily to the practice of meditation. Its premise is that the reader, having had an insight into the illusory nature of the ego, the transient, ephemeral world it projects, the restlessness and anxiety produced by its incessant desires and the activities undertaken to gratify them, its eternal promise of fulfillment that never becomes a reality, now wishes to be freed from its tentacles and consciously reestablish contact with Self.

Because of a number of prevalent misconceptions, it is important that the reader be aware of certain specific things

---

Yoga: The 8 Steps to Health and Peace. Richard Hittleman. Bantam Books, 1976.

that Yoga meditation is *not*. First, it is not prayer. For many people, prayer and meditation are interchangeable concepts. But prayer is the articulation of a particular thought that is usually supplicatory: it is the expression of a request, of gratitude, of repentance. This is not related to Yoga meditation. Second, widespread exposure to the techniques of psychotherapy has caused some people to think of meditation as a method of introspection in which one becomes involved with personality analysis and attempts to determine his "hang-ups," his positive and negative qualities so that he may function in a more complete, holistic manner and derive greater fulfillment from life. Again, such things are not a part of Yoga meditation. Finally, due to various gross distortions and misinterpretations, many young people have been led to believe that meditation is a vehicle for evoking a "blow-your-mind," "far-out" experience, a sort of sound and light show, a "trip" similar to that which might be induced by a drug. But to the serious student of Yoga meditation, these are totally alien objectives. In our meditation practice, nothing is articulated to deliberately activate the mind and emotions (supplication); no analysis is undertaken to reinforce and perpetuate the ego (introspection); no thrills or mystical experiences are intentionally sought. The objectives of Yoga meditation transcend all such ephemeral concepts; they pertain solely to *enlightenment* and *liberation*. It is with the application of those techniques which assist the student in achieving these objectives that this book is concerned.

Among those who become interested in meditation, reaction to a given technique can vary widely: some are attracted to it, others find it of little interest; for some it is highly effective in achieving a particular objective, for others it produces only minimal results. A *mantra* may seem to be an expedient technique, but in application a *yantra* can prove more effective. The student may find that he is able to quiet his mind through fixing his gaze on a flower, but he may also discover that the degree of quietude is significantly greater in Alternate Nostril Breathing. Deep Relaxation may appear to be exactly what is needed for revitalization, but in the course of practice, visualization of the White Light may produce better results. The point is that these things can only be determined by the individual student. Just as natural attraction and receptivity are critical factors in all things that people do, so are they major considerations in the practice of meditation. Therefore, the beginning student is best served by being exposed to and properly instructed in *a variety of classical techniques*. From such exposure, the student is able to determine the type of meditation practice to which he is attracted and receptive. He also gains a feeling of his ability to effectively apply particular techniques, and he notes his experiences with each. Through this process, the single technique best suited to his meditation practice will ultimately emerge.

The variety of techniques referred to above is presented in this *30 Day Plan*. I have been teaching these techniques for more than 20 years, and they have been used, in various forms, by untold millions of people over many centuries to achieve the objectives of meditation. The major objective for the beginning student is the quieting of the ordinary mind. (I employ the term "ordinary" to distinguish between the mind that "thinks"—the computer of the ego—and Universal Mind, which is pure, unconditioned Knowledge and Intelligence.) The consciousness will not turn inward as long as the agitation generated by ordinary mind (of which the senses are a part) persists. It is only when this agitation abates that we begin to perceive the state beyond ordinary mind. The traditional imagery describing this situation is that of the disturbance in a pool filled with pure, clear water. The ripples that form on the surface by any agitation of the water prevent one from seeing to the bottom of the pool; one sees only the ripples. But when they are stilled, visibility to the bottom is clear. The incessant activity of the mind and senses, generated by their preoccupation with the things and conditions of what appears as an external world, is comparable to the ripples that prevent us from seeing what lies beneath. Therefore, our primery concern is with controlling and quieting the ordinary mind. During the meditation session, we practice to achieve this control by deliberately restricting the movement of the attention. Utilizing the various techniques, we focus the mind upon a *single point* and attempt to hold it exclusively on this point for the indicated time. This steady, total fixation of the mind on a single point is designated the "one-pointed" state, and its attainment is essential for productive meditation.

The *30 Day Plan* is comprised of nine groups of meditation techniques; each group consists of two or more techniques. The course is progressive in the sense that each technique of a particular group is slightly more advanced than that which precedes it, or the same technique is slightly more advanced each time it appears. There is one technique for each of the 30 days, and the order in which they appear provides the variety of techniques and diversity of practices that make the student aware, on a daily basis, of the various dynamics involved in meditating. This arrangement also enables him to quickly develop aptitude in a number of critical areas during the relatively brief 30-day period.

The Plan includes the Hatha Yoga postures (*asanas*). The body and the ordinary mind are one entity. They exert a direct and constant influence on each other. When the mind is disturbed, a corresponding dis-ease manifests in the body. The converse phenomenon also occurs: a body that is ill-at-ease causes the mind to be even more agitated than it is in its usual restless condition. Because the *asanas* have an immediate quieting effect on not only the physical, but the subtle body, they can be of great assistance in helping the student to achieve that steady, one-pointed state which is essential for fruitful meditation.

The *asana* routines presented in this book have been especially designed as preludes to the daily practice of meditation and comprise an abbreviated course in Hatha Yoga. Those readers who are interested in a more detailed course in Hatha Yoga should see my books *Yoga: 28 Day Exercise Plan** and *Yoga: The 8 Steps to Health and Peace.* †

From time to time, I encounter a person who is attracted to the concept of meditation, but who thinks that various psychological and philosophical preparations are necessary before he can begin its practice. He will ask numerous questions concerning what he can expect from meditating; he states what he wishes to accomplish; he wants assurances and guarantees; he tells of the many difficulties (lack of time, discipline, facilities, and such) that prevent him from following through; he feels he must improve himself in other areas before he can begin meditating; he seeks to satisfy his intellect by detailed comparisons of the various systems of meditation; he is worried about possible religious or philosophical conflicts. All such things are totally unnecessary, constitute a tragic waste of time, and have nothing to do with the actual *practice* of meditation. If you want to learn what meditation is about, you must meditate. Now is the time to begin. Your age, background, beliefs, or current circumstances are irrelevant. If you can read the instructions in this book, you can meditate; your experiences in the course of practice will make clear the folly of those who hesitate and delay while they attempt to anticipate the meditation experience.

The next few pages inform you of the simple preparations necessary for productive practice. Read through them carefully and begin the Plan. There is nothing you could do during the next 30 days that would serve you to greater advantage.

*Workman Publishing Company, 1969. Bantam Books, 1972.
†Hittleman, *loc cit.*

Preparation
for Practice

Any clean, quiet indoor or outdoor area in which there is adequate ventilation and a totally flat surface will be suitable for practice of both the *asanas* and meditation. There must be sufficient light—natural or artificial—to see the book clearly. If you use a separate room specifically for your practice, furnish it gradually in a manner that you find conducive to quieting the mind and emotions. A partial area of a room can be similarly furnished. Whatever your arrangements, the major requirements for the practice area are that it is clean, flat, well ventilated and that the possibilities of being disturbed while practicing are minimal.

Each practice session will require approximately 20 minutes. Early morning is a good time for practice but, with the exception of the time immediately before retiring, any time is satisfactory. It is traditional to meditate at approximately the same hour each day. If you wish, you may practice twice on any given day. Use the meditation technique of that day for both sessions.

The special, abbreviated Hatha Yoga course for this Plan is progressive in that periodically, slightly more advanced positions of each posture are introduced. In relative terms, we may designate the three degrees of the positions "elementary," "intermediate," and "advanced." If you are unable to execute the more advanced positions of the postures at that point in the course where they appear, do not be concerned. *Never strain or experience discomfort in attempting to attain any of the positions.* Progress in Hatha Yoga must be gentle and gradual. When your body is ready, it will move into the next stage; if you strain in any way to prematurely advance, you will actually retard genuine progress. Therefore, it may be that at a later point in the course, you will be performing the more advanced positions of some *asanas* but still only the elementary positions of others. This is perfectly satisfactory. Simply continue to work gradually toward the advanced positions.

Once learned, each Hatha Yoga routine should require a period of 10 minutes. In the initial stages of learning, a slightly longer period may be necessary. When you become proficient in the movements, you may find them so enjoyable and beneficial that you may wish to extend the 10-minute period. However, during the initial 30 days of this course, the 10-minute periods are all that are mandatory. (If there is any concern regarding the physical effects of the Hatha Yoga routines, consult a physician prior to beginning their practice.)

If you have been using a Hatha Yoga practice plan from one of my other books, you can continue to do so. Any Hatha Yoga routine that has proven effective for you is satisfactory. You may substitute that routine(s) for those presented in this *30 Day Plan*. Simply add the meditation technique of the day to the end of the routine(s) you have been using. But remember that Observation of the Breath, as instructed in this course, must always immediately precede meditation.

If you choose to meditate twice daily, you need perform

the *asana* routine in one session only (it can be either session). Performing the *asana* routine in the other session is optional. If you are using a previous *asana* routine that is longer than those of this book, you may divide that routine between the two sessions. But remember that Observation of the Breath must precede meditation in both sessions.

• At least 90 minutes should elapse after meals before you begin either Hatha Yoga or meditation practice. Application of the Yoga Nutrition Principles is always advised.* The student should be aware of the effects of what he ingests. Avoid foods that excite, irritate, and cause various digestive disturbances. When the body is affected in this manner, corresponding disturbances are produced in the emotions and mind. Obviously, meditation is not assisted by such conditions.

Also in connection with disturbances, we must emphasize that indulgence in any and all consciousness-altering drugs is to be absolutely avoided. It is impossible to meditate in the manner prescribed in this book when under the influence of a drug, regardless of how benign that drug is believed to be. Certain of the effects produced upon the consciousness by various drugs are described by their users as "insight," "revelation," and even "enlightenment." But these are counterfeit experiences, illusions of the ordinary mind that soon vanish, having in no way furthered one in the objectives of quieting the mind and focusing it in the necessary one-pointed manner. Ultimately, drugs weaken and even destroy the will to devote the required time and energy to the practice session. Consequently, drugs (and, of course, alcohol) are incompatible with serious meditation. *There are no exceptions to this rule.*

• Practice clothing should permit complete freedom of

Yoga Natural Foods Cookbook. Richard Hittleman. Bantam Books, 1970.

movement. There must be nothing constricting on the body. Remove your watch as well as jewelry that is heavy or that interferes with the movements of the *asanas*. Glasses that are required for reading may be necessary, but remove them whenever they are nonessential for *asana* or meditation practice.

• A mat is needed. It should be 5–6 feet long, approximately 3 feet wide, and have a slight thickness so that it does not easily slip or wrinkle. This mat is used exclusively for your Yoga practice. It can remain on the surface of the practice area between sessions, but if there is the possibility of it being contacted by anyone (in walking, cleaning, and the like), then put it away following practice. Wash or clean it as necessary.

• A pillow that provides approximately 6 inches of sitting height may be helpful. (See instructions for the Cross-Legged Postures.)

• Place a timepiece that is silent and can be easily read in the meditation area. Do not wear it on your wrist.

• It will be necessary to continually refer to the book. At times you will need to hold it in your hands, and at times it must be at the correct distance to enable you to read instructions and see photographs for performing the *asanas* or for fixing and holding your gaze on the appropriate illustrations. Within a few days, you will be able to determine the best positions of the book for the various practices. To facilitate reference, adjustments may be made using a holding clip, paperweight, bookstand, and other types of support. Experiment with these.

• This course is comprised of a very carefully planned series of progressive steps. Application by the student of any other meditation techniques or procedures in conjunction with those of this book will conflict with its plan and impede the attainment of its objectives.

• At the conclusion of the 30 days, you will be advised to undertake Continuing Meditation by utilizing a limited number of techniques. This involves making a selection from those with which you have worked during the 30-day period. In this regard, having a brief summary of your experiences with, attraction or reaction to, and general impressions of each technique will prove valuable. Therefore, keep writing materials in your meditation area and, immediately following each session, note anything about your meditation practice that seems important. Recording this information on paper should require only a minute or two; you need not be overly analytical or become preoccupied with your literary style. If you feel that nothing of consequence has transpired, that too should be noted.

• If, on occasion, you are deeply absorbed in meditation and you sense that it is necessary to terminate the session, simply open your eyes and perform several deep breaths. Avoid the abrupt termination of meditation. If you are ever disturbed by anything external or internal that occurs during practice, open your eyes and quietly perform the breaths. When the interruption has passed, resume meditating.

• *I urge students not to discuss any aspects of their meditation practice with anyone.* Discussion of these matters is of no value and dissipates vital energies. The transformation of consciousness occurs in *silence.* Once you have begun serious meditation practice, this transformation process transpires even when you are not deliberately engaged in practice. It must not be intruded upon or disrupted through the ordinary mind's dissipative discussions and speculations.

• Make every effort to complete this course in 30 *consecutive* days. The consciousness will be transformed only by continually directing the mind inward. Although Self is our natural state, we do not recognize this fact without effort. The effort required is best put forth through *daily* practice. These daily sessions also build the momentum necessary to continue meditating on an extended basis following the initial 30-day period. If you do not establish and sustain the habit of daily practice, if your meditation is spasmodic, the impetus required to quiet the mind and turn it inward will be slow in coming.

• Do not anticipate results. The benefits derived from meditation are of an exceedingly subtle nature and do not manifest in the way that the beginner may expect. But they *do* manifest, and there is nothing in this life of which one is more acutely aware than such manifestations. What is required is that you be patient and regular in your practice. Realize that there is nothing you could be doing during the brief period you are devoting to meditation that would serve you to greater advantage.

Here is a summary of the regular items necessary for practice. Refer to the above pages for the details of each and for the conditions that should prevail in the practice area.

Appropriate clothing.

Mat.

A pillow is optional. You will make this decision in experimenting with the cross-legged postures.

Time piece.

A notebook and pen or pencil.

This book and whatever is necessary to position and support it for easy reference.

Using the Book

1. Having made the necessary preparations as described in the preceding section, sit down on your mat.

2. Take the book in your hands and refer to the appropriate day. You will note that each of the 30 days is divided into three sections:

> General information regarding the meditation technique of that day.
>
> The Hatha Yoga routine.
>
> Meditation practice.

Read the first section containing the general information. This general information appears at the beginning of the session and precedes the performance of the Hatha Yoga routine because actual meditation practice should immediately follow the *asanas* and Observation of the Breath. We do not want the meditation practice delayed any longer than is necessary to read the instructions for utilizing the meditation technique. After reading this first section, you will know the type of meditation practice with which you will be involved that day.

3. Look briefly at all the photographs for that day's Hatha Yoga routine. During the first week of practice, simply glancing at these photographs will assist in preparing you to perform the *asanas*. Later, this serves as a quick reminder of what is to be performed that day, and the body subconsciously readies itself.

4. Perform the Hatha Yoga routine to the best of your ability. Pay careful attention to all instructions; note particularly the emphasis on slow motion, graceful, nonstrenuous movements. You will have to continually refer to the photographs and instructions, so position the book accordingly. Each day's routine is terminated with Observation of the Breath, following which you proceed directly to the meditation practice.

5. Study the instructions and illustrations for meditation practice. There are several segments for each day's practice; whenever possible, memorize the instructions for all of the segments at the first reading. This way, you will not have to interrupt the continuity of practice with several readings. However, if you find such memorization difficult, you may read the instructions whenever you arrive at a point where this is necessary. Within a few weeks, you will probably develop the ability to retain the instructions for the entire meditation practice from the first reading. But because in both the *asanas* and meditation you must always be absolutely certain of how to proceed, it is far better to interrupt your practice at any point where you are uncertain of the correct procedure and refer to the instructions than to attempt to maintain the continuity and possibly proceed incorrectly.

6. Meditate with that day's technique exactly as instructed. With most techniques, it will be necessary to refer to the book; position it accordingly. Each day's meditation requires a period of 10 minutes. These 10 minutes are divided among

several segments of practice; the required time for each segment is specified in the instructions. However, we would like to avoid interrupting the meditation by having to periodically consult a timepiece in order to ascertain how much time has elapsed during a particular segment. Therefore, although various intervals of time are indicated for the segments, and a watch or clock appears in many of the meditation photographs, the specified time is best interpreted as approximate. You develop the ability to approximate 2 minutes, 5 minutes, and so forth. During the first few meditation sessions, occasional glances at the timepiece (which is positioned accordingly) will assist in developing such ability. It is simply a matter of cultivating the feeling of these various time periods, and this usually can be quickly accomplished. Once you are able to approximate the specified minutes, you can dispense with the timepiece.

We must also emphasize that the illustrations superimposed upon the photographs—those which depict the meditator's visualizations of the candle flame, the white light, the yantras, and the image of perfect health—are *approximations*. These illustrations are meant to convey to the student *approximately* how the images manifest with the *eyes closed*. However, there are differences among students in the way these images appear, and it should not be a matter of concern if the images that materialize in your visualizations differ in size or intensity from those depicted in the illustrations. What is important is that the general *form* of the image be as shown, and that you learn to visualize this form *continuously* during the meditation segment. The desired degree of intensity will come through practice. Any color or shade of black or white in which an image manifests is satisfactory.

7. Upon conclusion of the meditation session, take your writing materials (which have been placed in the meditation area prior to the beginning of the day's practice) and make whatever notations are pertinent.

Hatha Yoga

ELEMENTARY ROUTINE A

For Use on Days 1, 4, 7, 10

Be sure you have carefully studied
the information contained in the
Preparation for Practice section before
beginning the Hatha Yoga practice.

Pay particular attention to performing
the movements slowly, rhythmically,
gracefully, and without strain.

chest expansion

1. Stand with heels together, arms at sides. Interlace fingers behind back and *slowly* raise arms as high as possible without strain. Do not allow trunk to bend forward.

2. *Slowly,* without strain, bend backward several inches. You need not bend farther than position depicted. Look upward. Keep arms high and knees straight. Hold position without moving for a count of 5.

3. *Slowly* bend forward into position depicted. Do not go farther. Bring arms into indicated position. Neck is limp with forehead aimed at knees. Hold position motionless for a count of 10.

Keep hands clasped and *very slowly* straighten to upright position. Pause a few moments and repeat backward and forward bends. Straighten to upright position, unclasp hands, and gracefully lower yourself into a seated position on mat.

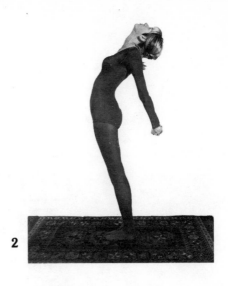

2

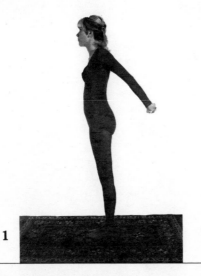

1

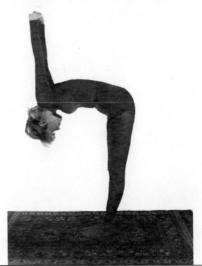

3

knee-and-thigh stretch

4. In a seated posture, place clasped hands around feet. (Trunk remains erect throughout the movements.)

5. Pull up against feet and slowly lower knees several inches toward floor. Hold without motion for 10. Relax

hands and allow knees to return to position of Fig. 4. Repeat. Perform 3 times.

Unclasp hands. Move gracefully into a lying position. Stomach and forehead rest on mat.

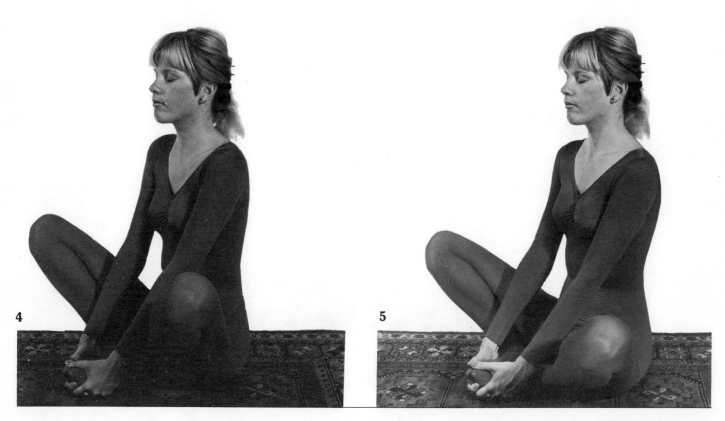

cobra

6. With forehead resting on mat, gracefully bring arms up from sides and place them beneath shoulders as illustrated. Note that fingers are together and point directly toward opposite hand.

In very slow motion, begin to raise head and bend it backward. Push against floor with hands and begin to raise trunk.

7. In very slow motion, continue to raise trunk. Head bends backward and *spine is continually curved.* Raise

trunk a moderate distance to approximately the position illustrated. Hold without motion for 10. Be sure that head is back and legs are relaxed during the hold.

In very slow motion, reverse the movements and lower trunk until forehead once again rests on mat. Relax a few moments and repeat. Perform 3 times. Relax with forehead on mat.

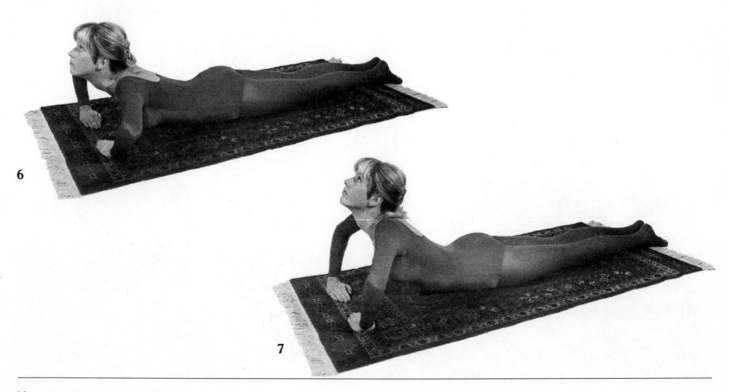

6

7

head twist

8. Remaining on stomach, raise head and place elbows on mat. Clasp hands firmly on back of head. Very slowly and gently push head down with hands until chin touches top of chest. Hold for 20.

9. Do not move arms. Turn head very slowly to left and rest chin in left hand. Grip back of head firmly with right hand. With the aid of both hands, very slowly turn head as far left as possible. Hold without motion for 20.

10. Do not move arms. Turn head very slowly to right and rest chin in right hand. Grip back of head firmly with left hand. With the aid of both hands, very slowly turn head as far to right as possible. Elbows remain on floor. Hold without motion for 20.

Repeat each of the three movements.

Rest chin on mat and lower arms to sides.

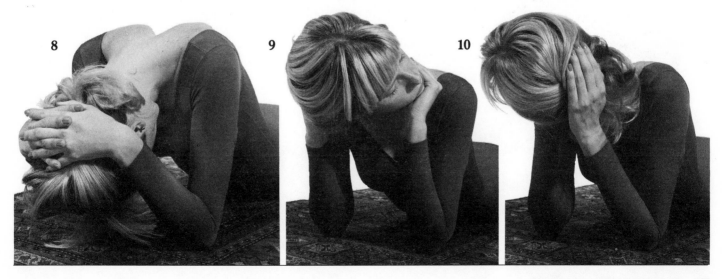

bow

11. Keeping chin on mat, hold feet as illustrated.

12. Slowly and cautiously raise head only. Pull hard against feet; raise trunk and knees a few inches from floor. Head is up, knees as close together as possible. Breathe normally. Hold without motion for 10.

Lower knees to floor, but retain hold on feet. Lower chin to floor and continue to hold feet. Pause a few moments and repeat. Perform 3 times. Following final repetition, release feet and lower them slowly to floor. Rest cheek on mat and relax.

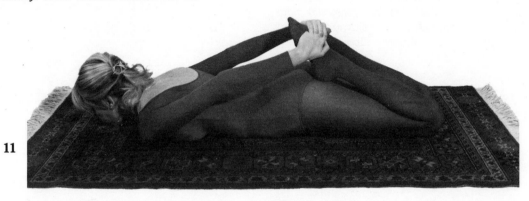

11

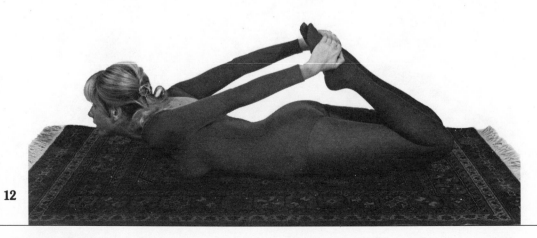

12

The Cross-Legged Postures

You will use one of the three cross-legged postures described below for the daily practice of *Observation of the Breath* and for all meditation techniques in which you are instructed to assume the cross-legged position. These are classical poses which have been used since time immemorial for the practice of meditation. Their value lies in the fact that when perfected, they enable the student to remain seated firmly, quietly, and alertly for the length of the meditation period. There are also esoteric ramifications that I have explained in my book *Yoga: The 8 Steps to Health and Peace.**

Although it is obvious that the Full Lotus is a more advanced position than the Half Lotus, and that the Half Lotus requires greater flexibility than the Simple Posture, we will not place these three in the "elementary," "intermediate," and "advanced" categories. From the very first day of practice, utilize whichever of the three you can assume without strain or major discomfort (the experiencing of some minor discomforts is usually necessary in the beginning practice of the cross-legged postures). If you choose to begin with the Simple Posture, continue to work toward the accomplishment of the Half Lotus. If you begin with the Half Lotus, work toward the Full Lotus. Through regular and patient practice, you gain the flexibility to execute the more advanced positions.

In each of the three postures, a pillow that provides approximately 6 inches of sitting height may be an asset in lowering your knees to the floor. Attempt the postures both with and without the pillow. If you conclude that it is helpful, place it in the practice area prior to your practice of the Hatha Yoga routines as it is used immediately upon completion of each routine for Observation of the Breath (performed in a cross-legged posture. In this book, the students depicted in the cross-legged postures are using pillows. The pillow is not used for any of the other seated *asanas*.)

If at any point during meditation in the cross-legged posture, you begin to experience the type of discomfort that proves distracting, do not endure this discomfort. Extend your legs and gently massage your knees and thighs for a few moments. Then resume the cross-legged position and continue your practice. Of course, this movement of your legs will disrupt your meditation, so it is important to develop the ability to remain in the posture, without discomfort, during the entire meditation period.

*Hittleman, *loc. cit.*

simple posture

13. Sit with legs extended.

14. Cross ankles (either one may be on top) and draw legs in as far as possible.

Trunk and head are erect but relaxed.

The backs of your hands rest on knees (or thighs), with thumbs touching index fingers and palms turned upward. There is slight pressure in the contact of the thumbs and index fingers, and this pressure is maintained as long as you are seated in the posture. This hand-and-finger position is a *mudra*.

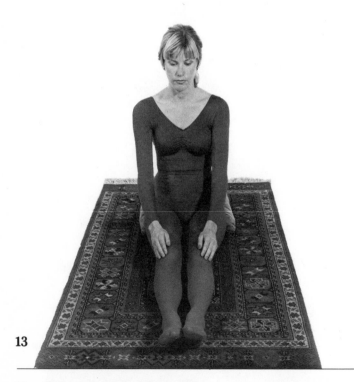

13

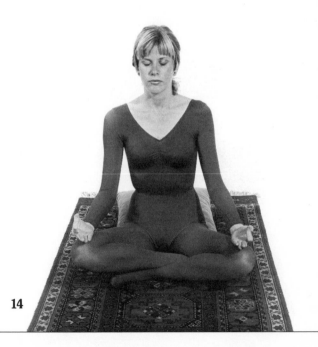

14

half lotus

15. Sit with legs extended.

Place left foot so that heel is as far in as possible.

16. Place right foot as high on left thigh as possible. Right heel is close to or touches groin. Trunk and head are erect but relaxed.

Execute the *mudra* as instructed in the Simple Posture. (The beginning student can practice the Half Lotus by first placing his right foot on top of his left thigh as instructed above, and then, when this becomes uncomfortable, exchanging the position and placing his left foot on top of his right thigh. However, he should concentrate on perfecting the traditional position, which is that of the right foot on top.)

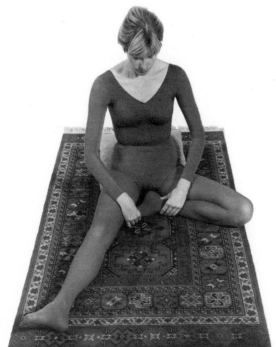

15

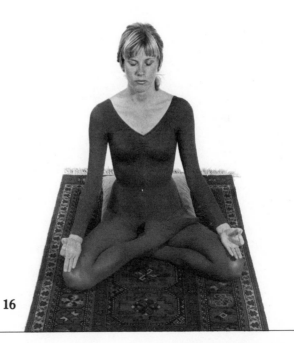

16

full lotus

17. Sit with legs extended.

Place right foot as high on left thigh as possible.

18. Place left foot as high on right thigh as possible. In the ultimate position of the Full Lotus, both heels press against groin. Trunk and head are erect but relaxed.

Rest hands on knees (or thighs) and execute the *mudra* as instructed in the Simple Posture.

(To aid in making his legs supple, the beginning student may also reverse their position. However, the position instructed above is the one to be perfected.)

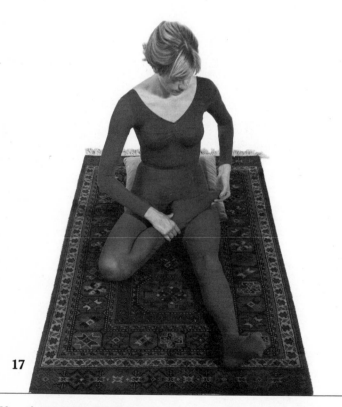

17

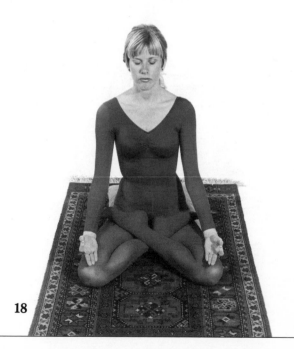

18

Observation of the Breath

This technique quiets the mind and senses and prepares them for the meditation practice that follows. Your breath is the source of your life. In observing the respiration process, you become consciously aware of that agent which is responsible for creating, sustaining, and ultimately terminating your life in this world. *Observation of the Breath directly precedes each day's meditation practice.*

19. Seated in one of the three cross-legged postures, direct attention to your breathing. Exclude all thoughts and sensations, and fix your consciousness totally on the process of respiration. Follow the air as it enters and leaves your nostrils and lungs. Become acutely aware of the inhalation and exhalation rhythm. Whenever this awareness is interrupted by a thought, a sound, and such, dismiss the interference and return attention to the breath. As often as you are distracted, you must return your attention to the breath. Observation of the Breath is continued for approximately 1 minute—just long enough to withdraw and quiet your mind and senses. According to the rhythm of your respiration, you will perform 9–15 inhalations and exhalations during the 1-minute period. (When the breathing is observed, its rhythm usually becomes slower.)

    Upon completion of this 1-minute preparatory technique, proceed with the meditation practice of the day.

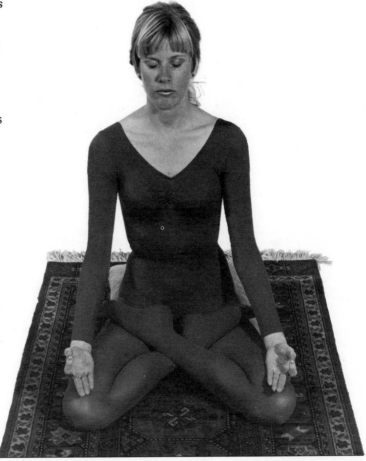

19

Hatha Yoga

ELEMENTARY ROUTINE B

For Use on Days 2, 5, 8, 11

rishi's posture

20. In a standing position, with heels together, slowly raise arms so that hands meet just below eye level. Fix gaze on backs of hands and very slowly turn trunk and arms 90 degrees to left.

21. Study illustration. Right hand moves slowly down inside of right leg and takes a firm hold on that area just below back of right knee. Left arm moves behind you to position illustrated, and gaze follows left hand.

Hold without motion for 10.

Slowly raise trunk to upright position and simultaneously bring arms back to extended position at eye level. Twist trunk to right and perform the identical movements on right side, exchanging the words "right" and "left" in the above directions. Perform 3 times to each side, alternating left-right. Following final repetition, slowly lower arms to sides and relax.

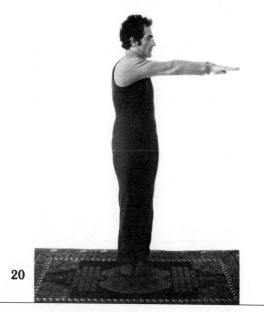

20

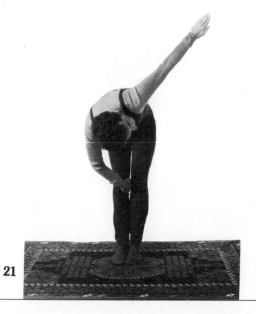

21

balance posture

22. With heels together, slowly and gracefully raise left arm straight upward.

Shift weight onto left leg. Bend right knee and raise right foot so that right hand can hold it.

23. Look upward and simultaneously pull right foot upward 1–2 inches so that you experience a gentle stretch in lower back. Hold as steady as possible for 5.

Slowly and gracefully return upraised arm to side, and foot to floor.

Now raise right arm and perform the identical movements with left leg. Hold position for 5.

Perform 3 times on each side, alternating sides.

Following final repetition, lower yourself gracefully into a seated position on mat.

(If you lose your balance at any point during the movements, pause a few moments and begin again. If you are unable to maintain or regain the balance after three attempts, proceed to the next *asana*. Balance will be gradually developed through repeated attempts.)

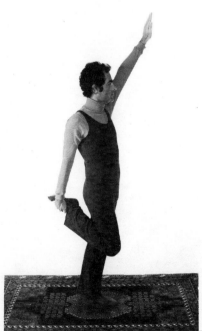

22

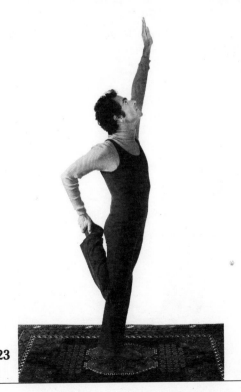

23

alternate leg stretch

24. Extend both legs straight outward.

Take hold of right foot and place right heel as high as possible against inside of left thigh. Right sole rests against (not under) left thigh.

In very slow motion, raise arms to overhead position. Look upward.

25. In very slow motion, with arms outstretched, execute a forward dive and firmly hold left calf with both hands. Lower right knee as far as possible toward floor. Back of left knee must be on floor.

Pull against left calf and, in very slow motion, lower trunk as far as possible without strain. Elbows bend

outward and forehead is aimed at knee. Hold without motion for 10.

Release calf and slowly straighten trunk to upright position.

Raise arms slowly and repeat the movements. Perform 3 times.

Following final repetition, straighten trunk to upright position, rest hands on thighs, extend right leg, place left heel against inside of right thigh, and perform the identical movements with right leg 3 times. Following final repetition, extend left leg (so that both legs are now extended) and rest hands on thighs.

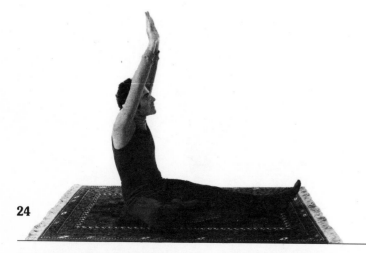

24

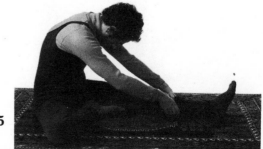

25

backward bend

26. Sit on heels. Knees are together.

27. Place hands on floor. Arms are close to sides. Slowly inch backward a moderate distance with hands. Note position of fingers: they remain together and point directly away from back. Slowly arch trunk upward and lower head backward, but remain seated on heels with knees together. Hold without motion for 10.

Raise head, relax trunk, and rest a few moments, but maintain position of arms.

Once again, slowly arch trunk upward and lower head backward, but remain seated on heels with knees together. Hold without motion for 10.

Raise head, lower trunk, and slowly move hands and trunk forward to starting position of Fig. 26.

Come off heels, swing legs around, and extend them straight outward.

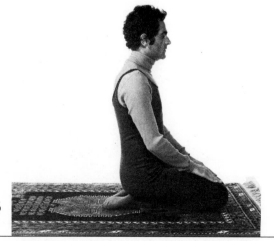

26

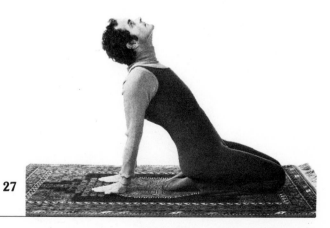

27

twist

28. Legs are extended.

Cross left leg over right leg and place left hand firmly on floor behind back.

Cross right arm over left knee and take a firm hold on right knee.

29. Very slowly twist trunk and head as far to left as possible. Hold without motion for 10.

Maintain position of hands, but slowly turn trunk frontward so that you are back in position of Fig. 28.

Relax a few moments. Repeat twisting of trunk and head as far to left as possible. Perform 3 twists.

Following final repetition, turn frontward, extend right leg, cross right leg over left leg, place right hand firmly on floor behind back, and perform the same twisting movements to right 3 times. (Remember to turn head as well as twist trunk.) Following final repetition, turn frontward, extend left leg, then assume cross-legged posture.

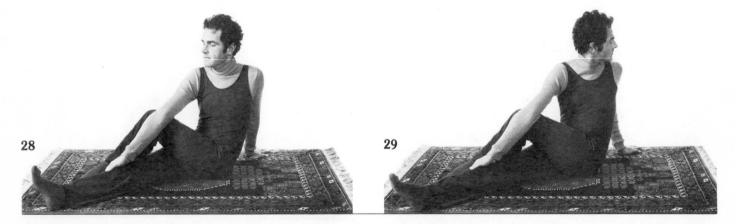

28

29

Observation of the Breath

30. Sit in cross-legged posture and observe the breath for
1 minute as instructed on page 21.

30

Hatha Yoga

ELEMENTARY ROUTINE C

For Use on Days 3, 6, 9, 12

triangle

31. Assume a stance with legs approximately 2 feet apart. Gracefully raise arms to shoulder level. Palms face downward.

32. Slowly bend to left and hold left leg just beneath knee. Pull on leg and lower trunk to approximately the position illustrated. Bring right arm (with elbow straight) over head to approximately the position illustrated. Hold for 10.

Slowly straighten to upright position of Fig. 31.

Execute the identical movements to right. Perform 3 times to each side, alternating left-right. Following final repetition, bring arms to sides, gracefully draw legs together, and lower yourself into a seated position on mat.

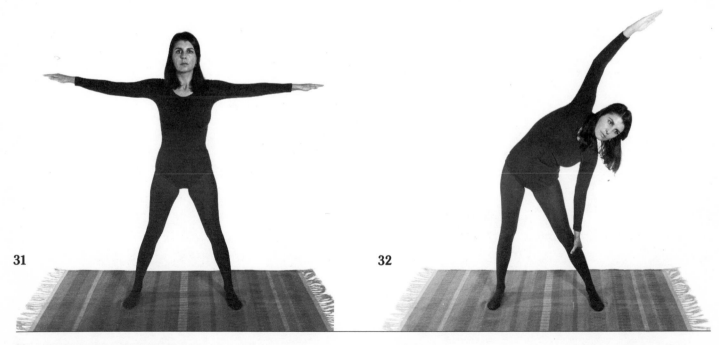

31

32

back stretch

33. Extend both legs straight outward. In very slow motion, raise arms to overhead position. Look upward.

34. In very slow motion, with arms outstretched, execute a forward dive and firmly hold both calves. Backs of knees must be on floor.

Pull against calves and, in very slow motion, lower trunk as far as possible without strain. Elbows bend outward. Hold without motion for 10.

Release calves and slowly straighten trunk to upright position. Raise arms slowly and repeat the movements. Perform 3 times.

Following final repetition, straighten trunk to upright position, rest hands on thighs, and slowly lower back to floor.

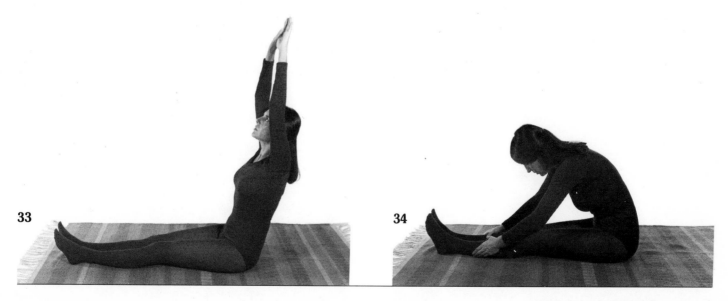

33

34

shoulder stand

35. In a lying position, place palms against floor and tense abdominal and leg muscles.

Press palms against floor and, with knees straight, raise legs slowly and bring them back gracefully over head.

36. Brace hands against hips and raise trunk and legs to position illustrated. Relax the body as much as possible. Breathe normally. Hold this position for 1–2 minutes. You may wish to use a watch for timing. If so, place it where you may see it easily from this inverted position. If you experience any strain or discomfort, shorten the length of the hold. If you are unable to raise your hips from the floor, simply raise your legs and hold them upright for the stipulated time. In some cases, swinging the legs back over the head with momentum will raise the hips so that the hands can be braced against them. Upon termination of the hold, slowly lower your legs behind your head for the Plough *asana*.

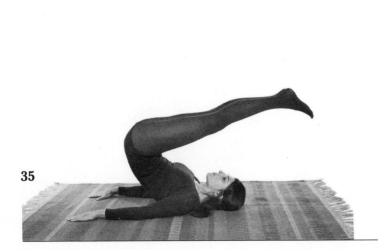

35

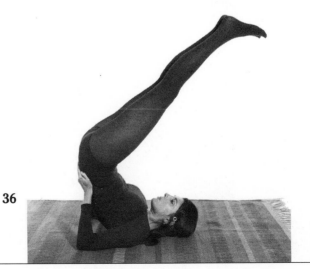

36

plough

37. From the Shoulder Stand position, slowly lower legs toward floor. Knees are held straight. When legs have been lowered a sufficient distance, you will be able to brace palms against floor.

38. Continue to lower legs (with knees held straight) until they are in approximately the position illustrated. Breathe normally. If position depicted is too difficult, simply lower legs as far as possible without discomfort, and continue to work toward the more extreme positions. Hold with as little motion as possible for 1 minute.

Come out of the position by bending knees and bringing heels to buttocks. Roll trunk forward slowly with as much control as possible, and attempt to keep back of head on floor so that trunk does not come lurching upward. When hips touch floor, extend legs straight upward and lower them slowly to floor. Relax a few moments in prone position and then come into seated cross-legged posture.

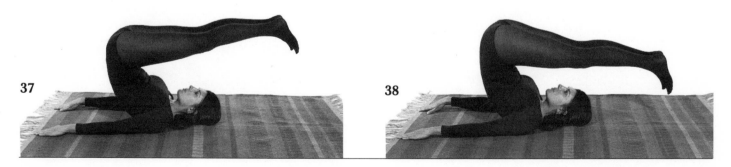

37

38

head roll

39. In cross-legged posture, close eyes, slowly bend head forward as far as possible, and relax neck. Hold without motion for 10.

In very slow motion, roll and twist head to extreme left. (Do not simply bend head to side; roll and twist it in slow, exaggerated motion.) Eyes remain closed. Hold without motion for 10.

40. In very slow motion, roll and twist head to extreme backward position. Hold for 10.

In very slow motion, roll and twist head to extreme right. Hold for 10.

In very slow motion, roll and twist head to original forward position. Repeat the four positions once.

Upon completion, remain in cross-legged posture, keep eyes closed, and raise head.

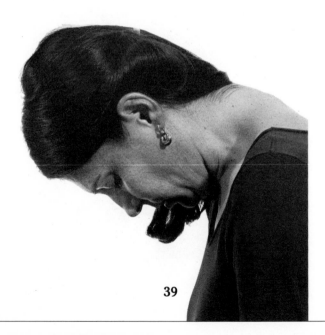

39

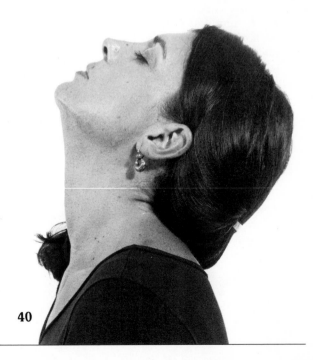

40

Observation of the Breath

41. Sit in cross-legged posture and observe the breath for 1 minute as instructed on page 21.

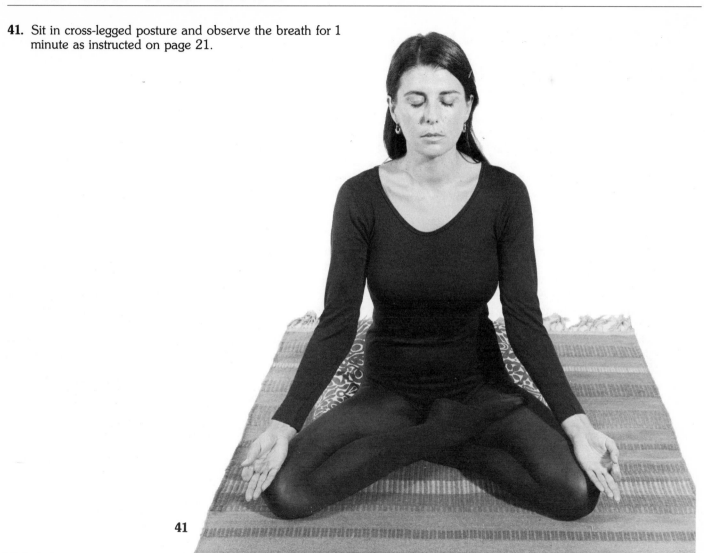

41

1st day

The Feeling of Deep Relaxation

It is now common knowledge that the mind has a profound influence on the body; various conditions that manifest in the body may often be directly traced to particular patterns of thought. But the converse is equally true: the condition of the body and the rhythm of the breath have an immediate effect on the emotions and the manner in which the mind functions. A person who is afflicted with anxiety, nervousness, and depression can frequently eliminate these and related conditions when he/she becomes sensitive to areas of tension in the body and learns how to deal with these tension patterns, learns how to "let go."

Although meditation is not to be equated with relaxation, it is true that when the body is tight, tense, uneasy, or agitated, productive meditation cannot be successfully accomplished. Even slight muscular contractions that frequently go un-noticed can impede the free flow of the required energy (*prana*). It is to eliminate these inhibiting conditions that we perform a routine of Hatha Yoga *asanas* prior to each meditation session. And today, in addition to these Hatha Yoga techniques, you will practice to not only deliberately place yourself in a state of deep relaxation, but to become acutely aware of the *feeling* of this totally relaxed state. The conscious feeling of this state is a profoundly important experience; it is an experience that only a relatively small number of people ever have. Its importance for students of Yoga and meditation lies in the fact that once recognized, once the *place* of that feeling is known, it can be contacted with increasing frequency. Eventually, the relaxed state become the *natural* state in which the student functions. The advantages of this condition in regard to health for the body and mind are obvious. What may be less obvious to the beginner is that a significant amount of *prana,* vital force, that is ordinarily dissipated in tension patterns can now be directed into concentrating the mind and helping to achieve that one-pointed state which is essential in meditation.

Each time this technique is practiced, a deeper stage of "letting go" will be experienced. There is a progressive unburdening of the body and mind which, coupled with other techniques that we apply, results in an indescribable state of lightness and freedom.

Instructions

Perform Hatha Yoga Elementary Routine A page 11

From the cross-legged posture, slowly extend your legs straight outward.

Slowly lower your back to the floor.

Place your arms as illustrated in Fig. 42. Palms face upward. Close your eyes. Breathe normally.

Allow your body to become limp.

Focus your full attention on your feet; if they are tensed in any way, relax them. Next become aware of your calves and knees, and relax them completely. Now determine if all muscles in your thighs and buttocks are relaxed.

Slowly draw your consciousness into your lower abdomen, then into your upper abdomen, then into your chest. As you become aware of each of these areas, make sure there are no muscular contractions.

Now shift your attention to your fingers, then to your lower arms, upper arms, and shoulders. Feel the condition of each of these, and withdraw all support so that they become totally limp.

Next determine if your neck is in a comfortable position; if not, adjust it. Finally relax your jaw and face.

Remain in this relaxed condition.

Fig. 42 depicts the body in a relaxed condition, but not totally so. The subject continues, unconsciously, to tense certain muscles. Frequently, in the first performance of Deep Relaxation, various contractions remain unnoticed. Therefore, having now achieved a general state of relaxation, it is advantageous to repeat the Deep Relaxation technique and "fine tune" this condition. During the second execution, the slightest contractions will be detected and the appropriate muscles relaxed. (Fig. 43 depicts the totally relaxed state.)

1st day

42. Attempting to relax, the student may be unaware that certain areas remain tensed. The arrows indicate points where contractions are frequently present and may go unnoticed during the practice of Deep Relaxation.

43. Total relaxation. The contracted muscles have been relaxed. The consciousness remains steadily focused on the *feeling* of this condition.

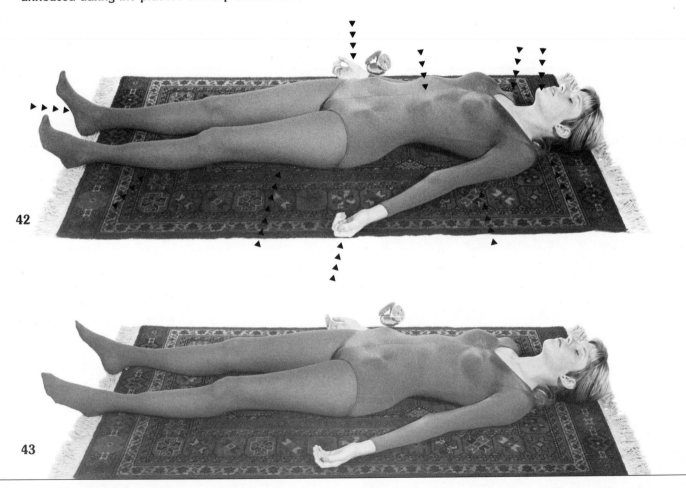

42

43

Once again direct your consciousness to your feet and proceed exactly as previously. With your attention now acutely focused on each area in turn, attempt to detect and relax all muscles that may have remained contracted, however slightly, in the first execution.

When your attention is focused in your facial area for the second time, approximately 5 minutes will have elapsed, and your body should be in the deeply relaxed state. During the next 5 minutes, become acutely aware of the *feeling* of this state. The point, or "seed," of this meditation technique is the total awareness of *how it feels to be deeply relaxed.* Whenever you catch your ordinary mind straying outward and beginning to entertain thoughts, immediately dismiss all such distractions and return your attention to the feeling. As often as your consciousness strays, it must be brought back gently but firmly to the feeling of the relaxed state.

When approximately 5 minutes have elapsed, open your eyes. Slowly raise your trunk and come into a seated position.

This terminates the meditation practice for today. (Make notes of whatever seems interesting, meaningful, important, and the like.)

(Tomorrow's meditation practice requires a candle and holder. Have these on hand for tomorrow's session.)

2nd day

Candle (1)

The ultimate state sought by the Yoga student—that of pure consciousness and unconditioned knowledge—is characterized in metaphysical literature with such expressions as "enlightened," "illuminated," "the mind is full of light, "the light penetrates the veils of ignorance." The element of *light* is repeatedly applied to the Self-realized state. The type of light that is involved cannot be accurately described because, in its brilliance and intensity, it transcends anything known through external vision. "Brighter than the brightest sun" is a phrase that is used. Because this internal light elevates, clarifies, and refines the consciousness, its generation is of great importance to the Yoga student. Our *30 Day Plan* includes several techniques in which light becomes the seed for meditation. Today's use of the candle provides the first such technique.

The flame of the candle has certain properties that make it particularly valuable for this practice of generating light. First, the eyes find it restful and interesting and are able to fix upon it with ease. Second, because of the nature of the impression that it makes upon the retina, it is relatively simple to retain. Therefore, the flame serves not only as an excellent introduction to visualization, but as that agent by which "the mind is filled with light."

Today's meditation requires a lighted candle. Place the candle (in its holder) and a match in your meditation area prior to beginning today's Hatha Yoga routine.

Perform Hatha Yoga Elementary Routine B page 23

Open your eyes.

Light the candle and place it approximately 3 feet from where you will be seated. Resume the cross-legged position.

Fix your gaze directly on the flame and hold it there steadily (blinking as necessary) for 2 minutes. Both your gaze and attention must remain fully fixed on the flame. If gaze remains fixed, but attention wanders, this technique will not produce the desired results. (Fig. 44.)

When the 2 minutes have elapsed, close your eyes and place your palms over them. (The candle remains lighted. See Fig. 45.)

With your eyes palmed, retain the image of the flame. It is usually a yellow-white color, although any color(s) in which it appears is satisfactory. Concentrate fully on that image for 3 minutes, and do not allow the flame to waver. If the image begins to fade, or if you lose it entirely, remanifest it by an intensified visualization effort. Each time the image fades, bring it back; each time you become aware that your attention has wandered, return it gently but firmly so that it is fully and exclusively occupied with the image. (If you lose the image entirely and find that you absolutely cannot remanifest it, open your eyes and fix your gaze on the flame for a brief period. Then palm your eyes and resume the practice.)

When the 3 minutes have elapsed, open your eyes. If you are experiencing discomfort in your legs, extend them slowly, massage knees gently for a few moments, and then resume the cross-legged posture.

2nd day

Repeat the procedure: gaze at the lighted flame for an additional 2 minutes; palm your eyes and retain the image of the flame for an additional 3 minutes. Remember that there is nothing to be done during the visualization period other than developing your ability in one-pointed concentration by occupying your consciousness fully and exclusively with the image.

When the 3 minutes of visualization have elapsed, open your eyes and slowly extend your legs. Extinguish the flame.

This terminates the meditation practice for today. (Make your notes.)

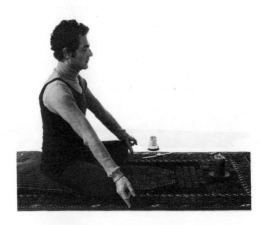

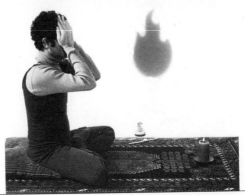

44. Full attention is focused on the flame for 2 minutes.

45. The eyes are palmed and the image retained for 3 minutes.

3rd day
White Light (Revitalizing)

Prana (life-force) is the subtle agent through which the life of the body is sustained. The more *prana* that enters and remains in the body, the higher the quality of life. A reduction in *prana* results in a lowering of vitality and a deterioration in the quality of life; when there is no *prana*, there is no life.

While food, water, and light are major sources of *prana*, the primary source is air. ("Life is in the breath.") It is during the process of respiration that *prana* collects in certain bodily centers, particularly the *solar plexus*, from where it is continually dispensed throughout the organism. When we experience negative physical and emotional conditions (tension, stress, illness, pain, depression, depletion of energy, and the like), it is possible to temporarily increase the volume of *prana* (through deep breathing), tap directly into the solar plexus—the major center where the increased *prana* accumulates—and direct this *prana* to that area of the organism where it is needed for therapeutic purposes.

Although the pranic current is invisible to the external eye, it is seen by the internal, subtle vision as a white light of great intensity. The visualization and direction of this white light, in conjunction with a particular method of respiration, is today's meditation practice. On this 3rd Day, we are emphasizing use of the white light, the pranic current, for *general revitalization* of the organism. On a subsequent day, we will apply the white light for *healing*. Thousands of Yoga students have quickly gained facility in making this a highly *effective* technique. Frequently, it produces excellent results the first time it is used. ·

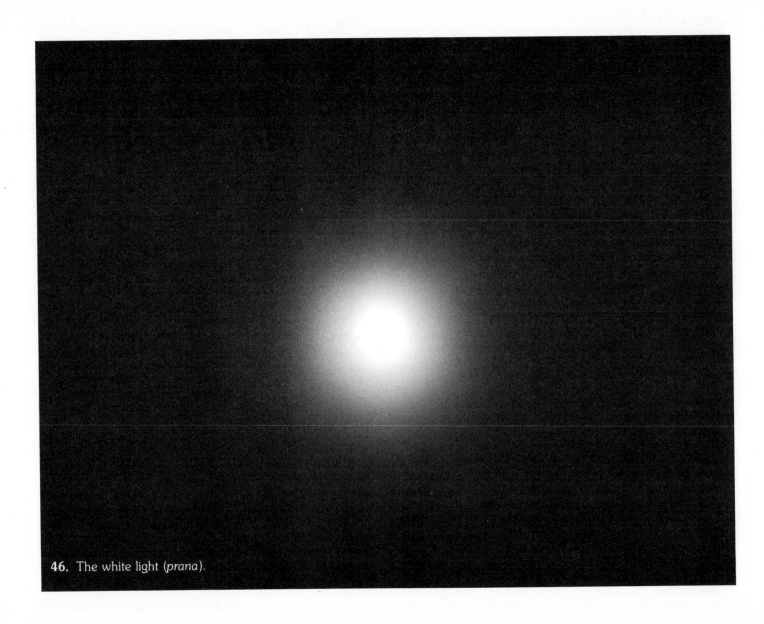

46. The white light (*prana*).

Instructions

Perform Hatha Yoga Elementary Routine C page 31

Remain in the cross-legged posture. Close your eyes.

The major center for the storage of life-force is the *solar plexus* (sun center). It is located at the top of the abdomen beneath the ribs. During respiration, *prana* collects in this area. Our objective today is to direct an increased supply of life-force into the head for purposes of calming and general revitalization.

Place all ten fingertips lightly on your solar plexus. Exhale deeply.

Very slowly inhale deeply and fully. During this inhalation, visualize the pranic current as an intense white light. (Fig. 46.) It enters through your nostrils, moves downward into the region of your solar plexus, and passes into your fingertips where it remains. This is the continuous visualization during the entire *slow* inhalation. (Fig. 47.)

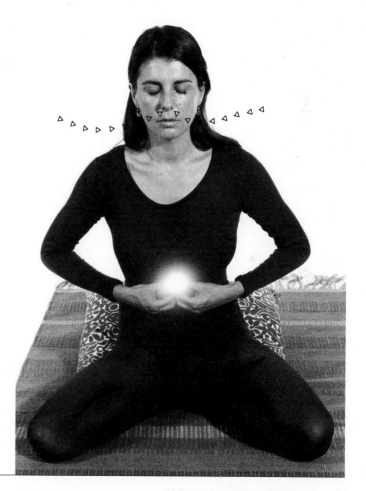

47. The course of the *prana* during the slow inhalation.

3rd day

When the inhalation is completed, *retain the air* and transfer your ten fingertips to the "third eye"—on the forehead between the eyebrows.

Very slowly exhale deeply and fully. During this exhalation, visualize the *prana,* the white light, flowing from your fingertips into your head, flooding it with life-force. This is the continuous visualization during the entire *slow* exhalation. (Fig. 48.) If your visualization of the white light flowing into your head is steady and strong, you will feel a pleasant tingling and warmth throughout your head. This sensation may extend to your body.

When the exhalation is completed, *suspend breathing* for a few moments while you slowly return your fingertips to your solar plexus.

Begin the inhalation and repeat the procedure.

During the 10-minute practice period, you will be able to perform approximately 20 repetitions. Obviously, your atten-

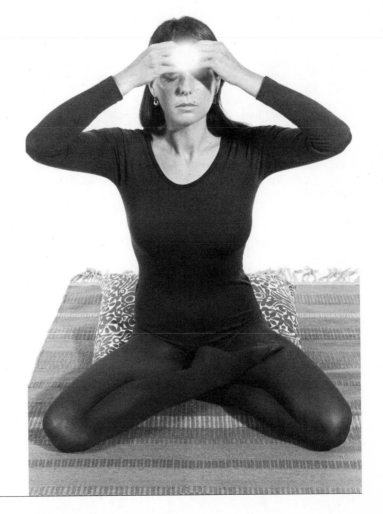

48. *Prana* is directed into the head during the slow exhalation.

tion must be fully focused on the visualization of the white light. If the light is slow in manifesting, persevere; it will come. If the white light fades, or is lost entirely, remanifest it by an intensified visualization effort. If your attention wanders, return it gently but firmly to the imagery.

When the 10 minutes of visualization have elapsed, keep your eyes closed, rest your hands (in the *mudra*) on your knees, and spend a few moments becoming acutely aware of what is transpiring within. (Fig. 49.)

Open your eyes and slowly extend your legs.

This terminates the meditation practice for today. (Make your notes.)

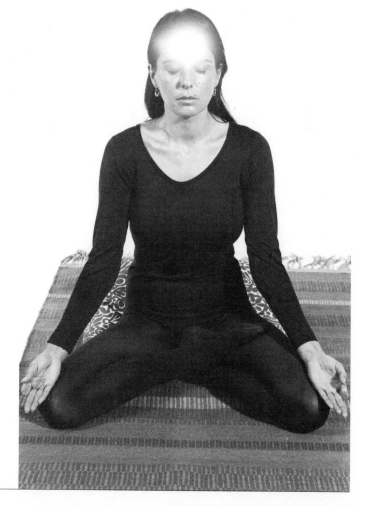

49. The increased supply of life-force remains in the head (and may be felt throughout the body).

4th day

Yantra (1)

To the casual observer, *yantras* may appear as little more than interesting designs, many of which, because of their use in various fields, seem familiar. For the Yoga student, however, yantras have the utmost significance: *they are mystical symbols of higher planes of consciousness.* When the meditator visualizes yantras in the prescribed manner, he becomes attuned to the vibrations embodied within them. Striking these sympathetic vibrations, his consciousness is drawn to those planes of which the yantras are graphic representations. With continued practice, the consciousness tends to remain longer and longer in this more rarified atmosphere where the intensified light illuminates one's vision and pierces those layers of darkness which obscure from him his true nature. Therefore, each contact with the higher planes refines the consciousness and increases one's understanding of Self.

Many yantras are universal; they are utilized as seeds for meditation not only in Yoga, but, with various modifications, in esoteric practices throughout the world.

Six yantras are utilized in this 30 Day course. Simple forms appear in the earlier sessions, and as the student's ability in visualization develops, more complex symbols are introduced. In the practice session, the student first absorbs the yantra through external concentration and then visualizes it internally.

Each yantra imparts its own unique form of energy, illumination, and refinement. With regular practice, the meditator will become sensitive to the value of a particular yantra as it relates to his personal development.

The dot within the circle, within the inverted triangle, is the yantra for today's meditation practice.

Perform Hatha Yoga Elementary Routine A page 11

Remain in the cross-legged posture. Open your eyes.

Place the book in a position where you may see it comfortably. (Fig. 50.)*

Fix your gaze on Fig. 51.

Hold your gaze steadily on the figure for 2 minutes. Both your gaze *and attention* must remain fully fixed on the figure. If gaze remains fixed but attention wanders, this technique will not produce the desired results.

Beginning at the top of the circle, direct your eyes slowly around the entire circumference in a clockwise direction.

*If you had to come out of the cross-legged posture to properly position the book, resume the posture before beginning meditation practice.

When you reach the 360-degree point, move your eyes into the center and observe the dot. Repeat this procedure for the 2-minute period.

Now close your eyes and visualize the identical figure for 3 minutes. Do not allow your attention to be diverted; no thoughts should enter your mind. If the image begins to fade, or if you perceive that your attention has wandered, re-manifest the figure by constructing the circumference of the circle in a clockwise direction and then placing the dot in the center. Any color in which the yantra appears is satisfactory.

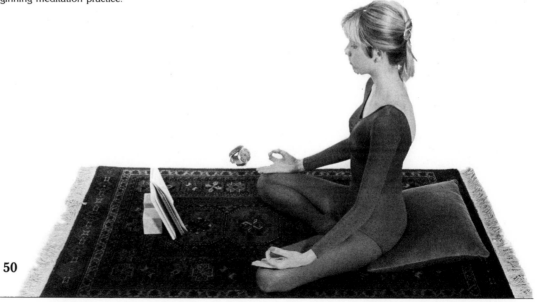

50

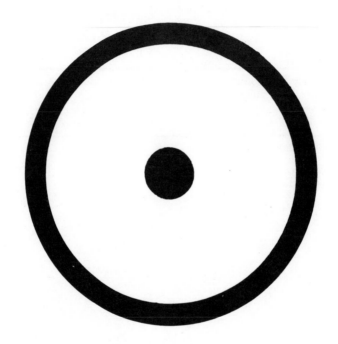

51. Yantra 1: the circle and dot.

When the 3 minutes have elapsed, open your eyes. If you are experiencing discomfort in your legs, you may extend them and gently massage your knees for a few moments. Then resume the cross-legged position.

Fix your gaze on Fig. 53. You will note that the yantra is now encompassed by an inverted triangle. Hold your gaze steadily on this figure for 2 minutes.

When the 2 minutes have elapsed, close your eyes and visualize the identical figure for 3 minutes. Again, do not allow your attention to wander. If the image fades, remanifest it by constructing the inverted triangle (beginning at the bottom point and moving clockwise to draw the three sides), then the clockwise circle within the triangle, then the dot.

If, during your initial attempts, the visualizations are impossible or extremely weak, reinforce the image by opening your eyes and observing the figure on the page for a brief period. Then close your eyes and make another attempt. By continuing to do this, your visualization ability will develop.

When the 3 minutes have elapsed, open your eyes and slowly extend your legs.

This terminates the meditation practice for today. (Make your notes.)

52. The simple (left) and more complex yantras are visualized successively.

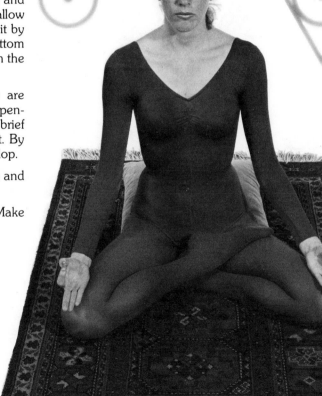

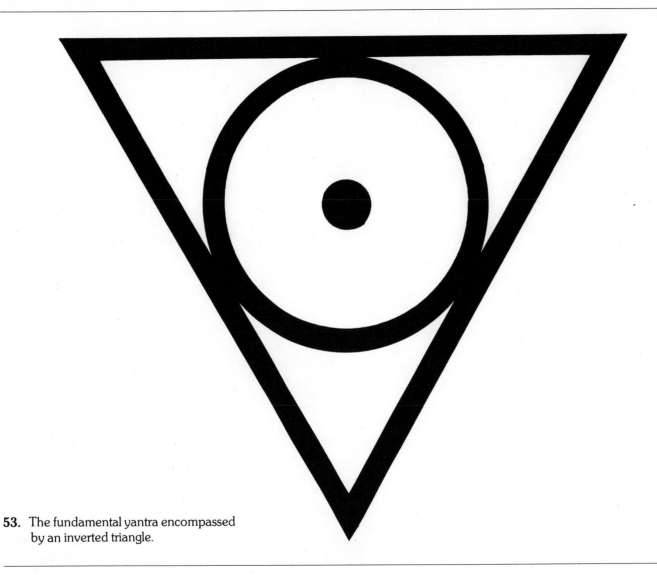

53. The fundamental yantra encompassed by an inverted triangle.

5th day

Alternate Nostril Breathing (1)

Everywhere in the external world we encounter manifestations of the positive-negative principle: in the composition of the atom, in the cell, in the polarity of the earth, in the sun-moon relationship, in the existence of man-woman. In those dimensions of existence which we gradually come to perceive through our inner vision, the same positive-negative phenomenon occurs. And just as in the external world we know that a certain balance must always be maintained in the positive-negative ratio, so it is that in our subtle, etheric bodies, a balance must be maintained in the constant interplay of positive-negative pranic current. We have already implied in the text of the White Light (3rd Day) that a reduction or imbalance in the flow of *prana* is responsible for physical, emotional, and mental disturbances.

The value of Alternate Nostril Breathing for the student of meditation lies in the fact that *it produces an automatic quieting of the mind.* Without any special effort other than the proper execution of the exercise, the mind and senses are profoundly relaxed. This relaxation is the natural result of having at least temporarily achieved a state of balance in the positive-negative ratio of the *prana* that enters the body through the respiration process. With the mind and senses in this deeply relaxed and quiet state, a remarkable insight occurs: the student begins to perceive that his true nature, that which he really IS, lies beyond the positive-negative condition, beyond all duality. This Truth can only be understood in total Stillness. To paraphrase Patanjali, the great synthesizer of Yoga practices: When the movements of the mind are restrained, Yoga is achieved. We can cultivate this restraint by eliminating the agitation that is produced when the positive and negative forces are unbalanced. Alternate Nostril Breathing is so effective in accomplishing this objective, we devote 4 of our 30 meditation sessions to its practice. In each of the three subsequent sessions, the rhythm of the breathing is modified from that of today because the depth of the relaxation and quietude can be gradually increased through these modifications.

Perform Hatha Yoga Elementary Routine B page 23

54 – Remain in the cross-legged posture with your left hand
55. in the *mudra.* Keep your eyes partially closed (only a
slit of light should enter at the bottom).

Place the tip of your right thumb lightly against your right
nostril and your ring and little fingers lightly against your left.
Your index and middle fingers are together, and they rest
lightly on your forehead (the "third eye" area).

Slowly and as quietly as possible, exhale deeply through
both nostrils.

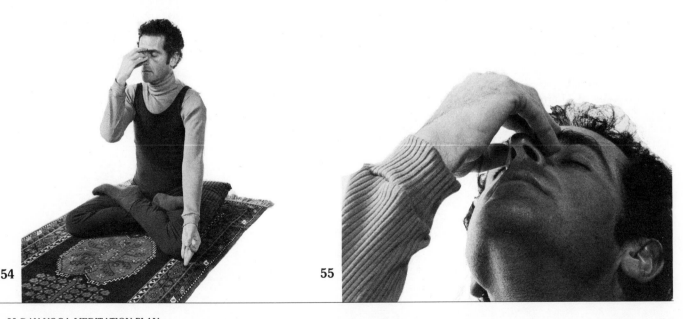

54

55

56. When the exhalation is completed, immediately close your right nostril by pressing your thumb against it. Slowly and quietly inhale deeply through your left nostril during a rhythmic count of 8.

57. Keep your right nostril closed and now press your left one so that both are closed. Retain the air for a rhythmic count of 4.

58. Release your right nostril (your left one remains closed) and exhale slowly, deeply, and quietly during a rhythmic count of 8.

57

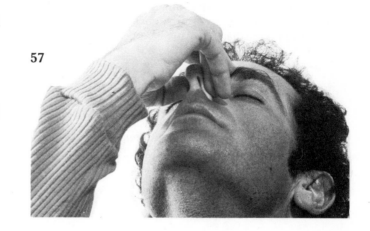

56

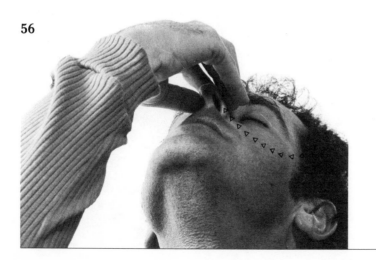

58

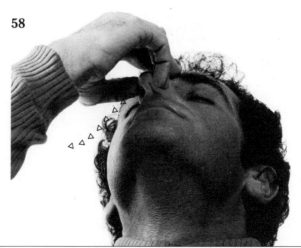

5th day

59. When the air is completely exhaled, do not pause; immediately begin the next inhalation through your *right* nostril (the same nostril through which you just completed the exhalation). Inhale a deep, quiet breath through your right nostril during a rhythmic count of 8. Your left nostril remains closed.

60. Keep your left nostril closed and now press your right one so that both are closed. Retain the air deep in your lungs during a rhythmic count of 4.

61. Release your left nostril (your right one remains closed) and exhale slowly, deeply, and quietly during a rhythmic count of 8.

60
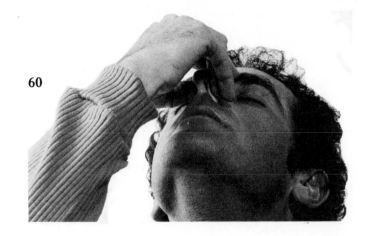

59
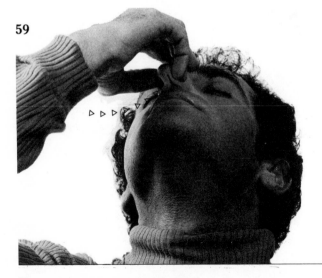

61
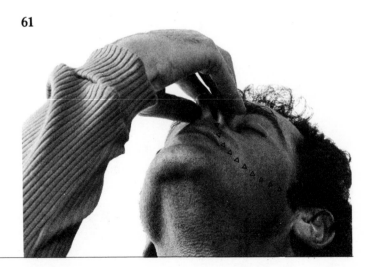

You have now returned to the original starting point. Each time you return to this starting point, you have performed 1 complete round of Alternate Nostril Breathing.

Without pause, keep your right nostril closed and begin the next round with a deep, quiet inhalation through your left nostril during a rhythmic count of 8.

Perform 7 rounds.

62. Lower your right hand and place it (in the *mudra*) on your right knee (or thigh).

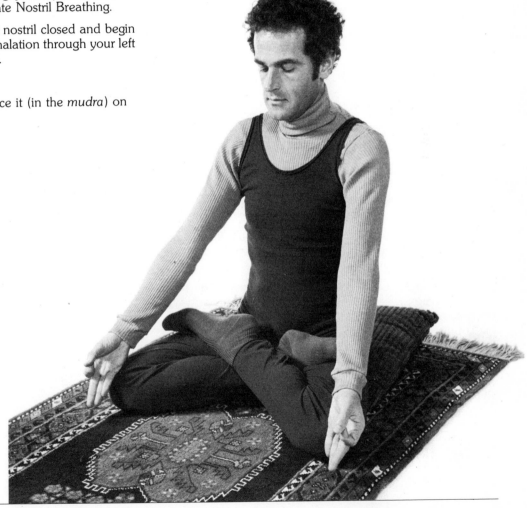

62

5th day

Summary

inhale through left	count 8
retain; both closed	count 4
exhale through right	count 8

without pause

inhale through right	count 8
retain; both closed	count 4
exhale through left	count 8

This completes 1 round. Without pause, begin the next round.

Do not permit your breath to gush or hiss in or out. Perform the inhalations and exhalations as quietly as possible. Think of the breathing as occurring more in the throat than the nostrils.

The counting is rhythmic and continuous; it is never interrupted. Once the counting begins, you keep it going like a metronome, steady and rhythmic.

Throughout the exercise, your attention must be fully focused on the counting. It must not become automatic while your attention is allowed to wander. Total concentration on the counting, in conjunction with respiration, is the seed for this meditation practice.

When you have completed the 7 rounds, remain seated quietly for a short interval, and become aware of the serene, elevated state of your consciousness. (Fig. 62.)

Open your eyes and slowly extend your legs.

This terminates the meditation practice for today. (Make your notes.)

6th day

OM (1)

A *mantra* is a special sequence of Sanskrit letters and syllables. Just as yantras are *symbols* of higher planes of consciousness, so are mantras the *sounds* of these planes. What the yantra effects through form and visualization, the mantra effects through a sequence of sounds. The student intones the mantra (audibly or silently) according to the prescribed rhythm and number of repetitions so that he may absorb its vibrations. His objective is to effect Yoga (fusion) with the sound that is generated.

Most mantras that are currently utilized have ancient origins. The supreme mantra that can be intoned to great advantage by all students is the sound produced by A-U-M. The eternal cycle of the day and night of Brahma—the cycle of creation, preservation, dissolution, and silence—is represented by A as the first sound (the creation), U as that of preservation, and M representing dissolution. The actual pronunciation is "Oh-Mmm." Therefore, Brahma, the Absolute Itself, is the essence of this supreme, all-encompassing mantra. OM is the word that generates those vibrations which form, sustain, and dissolve all things; OM is the universal sound that underlies all phenomena, gross and subtle, and it is heard in the state of Silence. By intoning this supreme mantra, the aspirant places himself in concert with the eternal cycle. (". . . the Word was with God, and the Word *was* God.")

The OM mantra is a classical and basic seed for meditation. Its intonation imparts a profound sense of quietude and elevation.

Perform Hatha Yoga Elementary Routine C page 31

Remain in the cross-legged posture. Your eyelids are partially lowered.

Exhale deeply.

In a count of 4 (approximating seconds), inhale deeply and quietly.

We will now intone OM (pronounced as it is in "home"). In a firm, steady, controlled voice, produce the sound "Oh" from the *back* of your mouth. (The lips are in the form of an "o." See Fig. 63.) This should be performed in a count of 2 (approximating seconds).

Without interruption, continue the "Oh" sound, but now let it proceed from the *front* of your mouth. As it moves to the front, it becomes slightly nasal in character. (The lips remain in the "o" shape. See Fig. 64.) This second sound is also performed in a count of 2.

Without interruption, press your lips together and produce the sound "Mmmm." (Fig. 65.) This sound should resonate strongly, like the buzzing of a bee, and you should feel the vibrations throughout your head and chest. Perform this in a count of 4.

Keep your lips together and *silently* complete the exhalation so that your lungs are emptied during an additional count of 2.

Without interruption, inhale deeply and quietly in a count of 4.

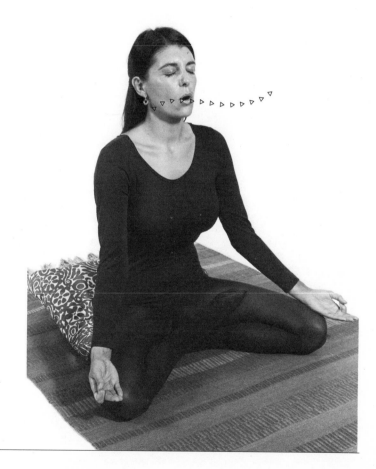

63. The "Oh" sound proceeds from back of mouth; lips in "o" shape.

64. "Oh" sound is transferred to front of mouth and has slight nasal quality; lips remain in "o" shape.

65. Lips together; strong vibrations of "Mmmm" throughout head and chest.

66. The attention is fixed on what is transpiring within.

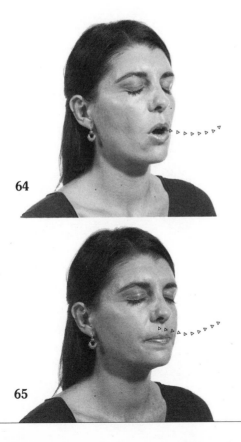

64

65

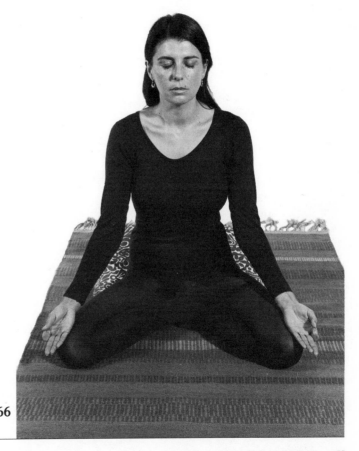

66

6th day

Repeat the mantra. (Repetition of a mantra is known as *japa*.) Devote 5 minutes to *japa*; you will be able to perform approximately 20 repetitions during the 5-minute period. (See Summary below.)

When the 5 minutes have elapsed, sit very quietly for another 5 minutes and become aware of what is transpiring within. Focus your attention fully on what you are experiencing, and do not allow your mind to wander.

When the 5 minutes have elapsed, open your eyes and slowly extend your legs.

This terminates the meditation practice for today. (Make your notes.)

Summary

	Deep inhalation	"Oh"	"Oh"	"Mmmm"	Finish exhalation
Sound characteristics	Silent	Proceeds from back of mouth; lips in "o" shape	Transferred to front of mouth; has slight nasal quality; lips remain in "o" shape	Lips together; strong resonance vibrating throughout head and chest	Silent
Time (attempt to approximate seconds)	4	2	2	4	2

The rhythm remains steady: an uninterrupted 4, 2-2-4, 2.
Fix this rhythm firmly in your mind before beginning the practice.

The voice is steady, firm, controlled, and remains on the same pitch.

The attention if fully focused on the sound. You must not allow the *japa* to become automatic while your mind and senses wander.

7th day

Asana Meditation (1)

In the first stages of Hatha Yoga practice, the student's attention is fully occupied with the dynamics of *learning* the movements. Except for the slow-motion approach, many beginners do not detect the differences between the Yoga *asanas* and the ordinary, calesthenic-type exercises. Once learned, however, not only does the student begin to experience the unique effects of the Hatha Yoga routines, but he learns how his mind may be directed to increase their effectiveness. This special direction of the mind becomes a form of meditation, and each *asana* is a seed for meditation. For the more advanced student, the entire Hatha Yoga session, from the first to the last movement, is a meditation practice.

As of today, you will have performed the *asanas* of Routine A three times, and be sufficiently familiar with their movements to utilize them as seeds for meditation. An *asana* is converted from a physical exercise to a meditation practice in the following manner: the attention is fully focused on the movements; the mind is no longer occupied with simply executing the movements, with *doing* the exercise, but becomes totally immersed in the *feeling* of the movements and aware of their effects on the areas of the body that are involved. This feeling technique is particularly applicable during the hold segment of the *asana*. When you are in your extreme position, and holding this position without movement, your attention is directed to that area of the body where the maximum stretch, pull, weight, and such is experienced. This focusing on the feeling of the emphasized area stabilizes and calms the mind and, through intense concentration, accelerates progress in the *asanas*.

The instructions for applying this technique to Routine A appear in today's meditation text. To reinforce the value of focusing the attention in this manner, we will have similar sessions with Routines B and C on subsequent days. Upon completion of the 30 Day course, you will be advised to utilize this technique in each of your Hatha Yoga practice sessions.

Perform Hatha Yoga Elementary Routine A page 11

Repeat the identical routine of Hatha Yoga *asanas* that you performed today. The postures will now be performed *with your total attention focused on all of the movements.* You are to *feel* their effects on the areas of the body that are involved.

The arrows indicate those particular areas of the body which receive the greatest emphasis during the hold. Direct your consciousness to the indicated area and maintain it there for the duration of the hold. If you detect that your attention is wandering, return it immediately to the movements or the hold.

Rest briefly between *asanas*. The number of repetitions for the *asanas* in this meditation routine differs from that of the regular routine.

Now stand up gracefully, turn your attention inward, and perform the routine.

67. The backward bend position. Hold for 10.

68. The forward bend position. Hold for 20.

69. Hold for 20. Perform twice.

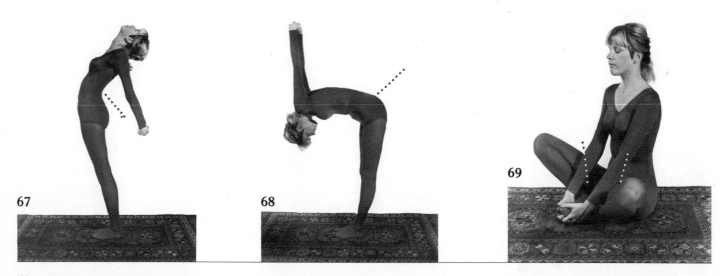

67

68

69

70. Hold for 10. Perform twice.

71. Hold each of the three positions for 20.

72. Hold for 10. Perform twice.

Upon completion of the routine, assume the cross-legged posture and rest for approximately 1 minute with your eyes partially closed. Become aware of how your body feels at this point.

Open your eyes and slowly extend your legs.

This terminates the meditation practice for today. (Make your notes.)

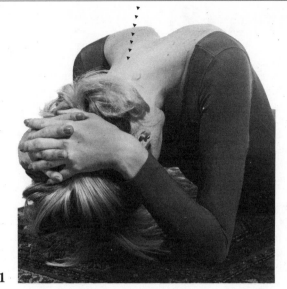

71

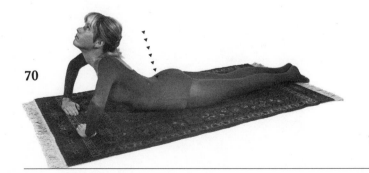

70

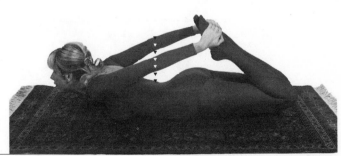

72

8th day

Yantra (2)

The second of the yantras for meditation is the cross. We utilize the cross that is formed by two intersecting lines, crossing at their midpoints. Embellished in various ways, this ancient mystical symbol is found in the literature and practices of esoteric organizations throughout the world. It has been recognized over the ages as a graphic representation of a higher plane of consciousness. It is to establish contact with this plane, to become attuned to its vibrations, and, eventually, to merge with it that we impress its representative yantra upon our consciousness.

As with the previous yantra—the dot within the circle—this yantra is visualized first in its fundamental form (the cross) and then in a more complex form (encompassed by a circle).

Be patient if your visualization attempts do not meet with complete and instant success. For the beginner, there is significant value to be derived from absorbing the energies of the yantra through the simple expedient of fixing the gaze upon the figure. The more advanced technique—visualization—is developed through practice.

Perform Hatha Yoga Elementary Routine B page 23

Remain in the cross-legged posture. Open your eyes.

Place the book in a position where you may see it comfortably. (Fig. 73.)* Fix your gaze on Fig. 74.

Hold your gaze steadily on the figure for 2 minutes. As previously, both your gaze and attention remain fully on the figure.

*If you had to come out of the cross-legged posture to properly position the book, resume the posture before beginning meditation practice.

Direct your eyes slowly from the top of the vertical line to the bottom, then from the left side of the horizontal line to the right. Repeat this procedure for the 2-minute period.

Now close your eyes and visualize the identical figure for 3 minutes. Do not allow your attention to be diverted; no thoughts should enter your mind. If the image begins to fade, or if you perceive that your attention has wandered, re-manifest the figure by constructing the vertical and horizontal lines.

When the 3 minutes have elapsed, open your eyes.

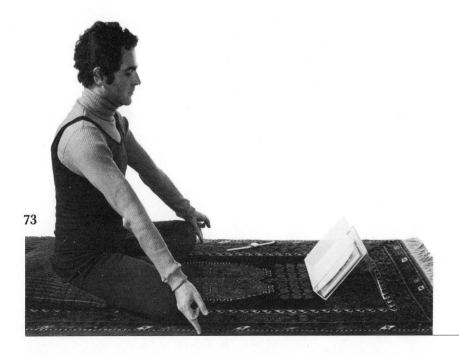

73

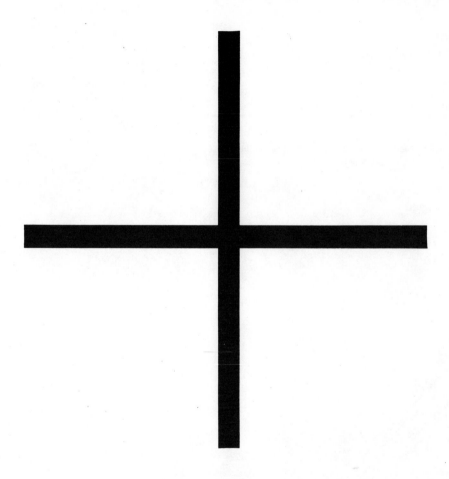

74. Yantra 2: the cross.

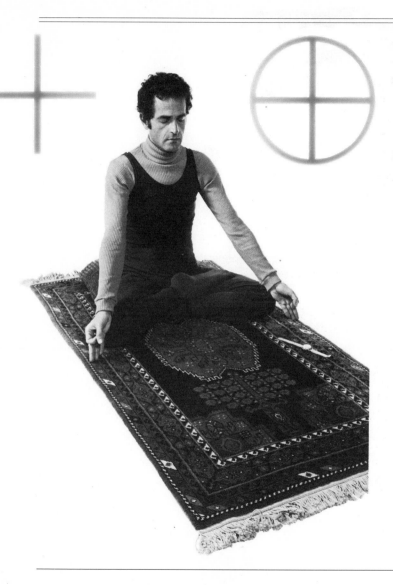

Fix your gaze on Fig. 76. You will note that the cross is now encompassed by a circle. Hold your gaze steadily on this figure for 2 minutes.

When the 2 minutes have elapsed, close your eyes and visualize the identical figure for 3 minutes. Again, do not allow your attention to wander. If the image fades, remanifest it by constructing the vertical and horizontal lines of the cross and then encompassing the cross with a clockwise circle.

If you are still finding the visualizations weak, reinforce the image by opening your eyes and observing the figure on the page for a brief period. Then close your eyes and make another attempt. By continuing to do this, your visualization ability will develop.

When the 3 minutes have elapsed, open your eyes and slowly extend your legs.

This terminates the meditation practice for today. (Make your notes.)

75. The simple (left) and more complex yantras are visualized successively.

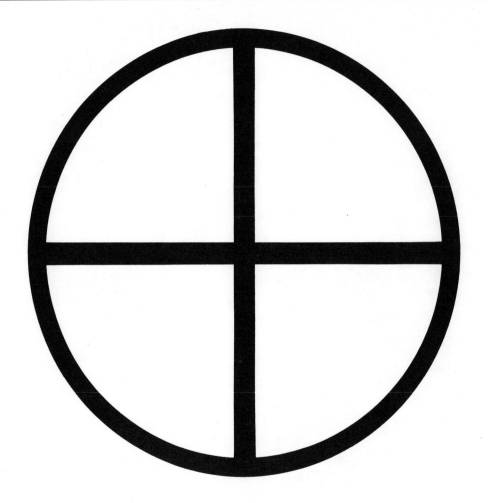

76. The fundamental yantra encompassed by a circle.

9th day

Active Meditation (1)

Today's meditation is described as "active" because there is a simultanaeity of imagery and body motion. Utilizing an *asana* in conjunction with a particular method of breathing (the Complete Breath), we *feel* and *visualize* a continuous, smooth progression from the passive to the active and back to the passive state. This pattern represents growth and decay, expansion and contraction, gain and loss; it is symbolic of the cycle that is inherent in all things manifest in the universe.

Injecting ourselves consciously into this cycle and experiencing its rhythm in an abbreviated and intensified manner helps promote our understanding of the condition that prevails in all aspects of life. When we have this direct awareness of how the principle of duality dominates our lives, we develop the perspective not only to deal with our ups and downs in a dispassionate manner, but we become convinced of the value of transcending the opposites and integrating with that principle from which duality arises. Integration with the principle beyond duality—the ONE—is Yoga.

Perform Hatha Yoga Elementary Routine C page 31

The *asana* performed in Active Meditation is the Complete Breath Standing.

Come into a standing position.

77. Exhale deeply and allow your trunk to relax as depicted. This stance represents an attitude of depletion. A minimum of life-force is present. Feel and visualize this passive state. (Your eyes are partially closed and can remain this way through the *asana*.)

78. Begin a very deep, very slow inhalation. As you inhale, expand your abdomen to permit the air to enter your lower lungs.

Begin to raise your arms slowly, palms up. As life-force (*prana*) enters your lungs, the organism is activated and stirs. Feel and visualize this birth of activity.

79. Continue the deep, slow inhalation and the slow raising of your arms with your elbows straight. (If the inhalation is not performed very slowly and very deeply, it will be completed before you can perform the necessary physical movements.) Now your chest expands, and as more air enters your lungs and more life-force fills your body, you become increasingly alive.

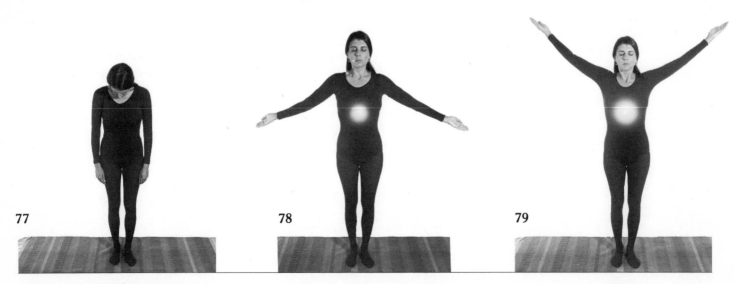

77 78 79

80. As your palms meet overhead, the inhalation is completed. Your lungs are full, your chest is expanded, your abdomen is slightly contracted. Retain the air for a count of 5. Feel and visualize your body permeated with *prana* and totally vitalized.

81. Begin a very slow exhalation. The movements are now reversed. Your arms are slowly lowered, palsm turned down. As the exhalation continues, the life-force is gradually depleted, and your trunk becomes increasingly limp. Feel and visualize this progressive depletion. (If the exhalation is not controlled, it will be completed before you have had the opportunity for adequate visualization.)

When the exhalation is completed, your arms rest once again at your sides, and the organism should be felt and visualized in the depleted, passive state. Suspend your breath so that no air enters your empty lungs for several seconds. (Fig. 77.)

Repeat the *asana*. Devote 5 minutes to Active Meditation. During this period, you will perform approximately 8 repetitions. The movements of the *asana* are simple, and you will be able to learn them in the first few repetitions. Thereafter, your attention must be fully focused on the feeling and visualization of the passive-active-passive-active dynamics.

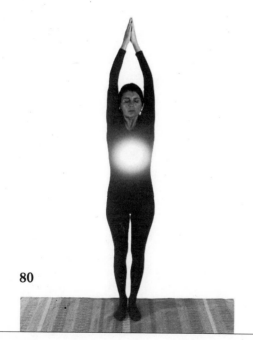

80

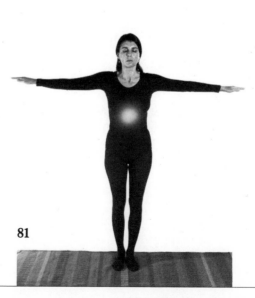

81

9th day

At the end of the 5-minute period, lower yourself gracefully to the floor and assume the cross-legged posture. Close your eyes.

For the remaining 5 minutes of the session, and for the only time in this 30 Day course, we encourage the ordinary mind to engage in the thinking process as a meditation technique. Contemplate the way in which the positive-negative principle is prevalent in all aspects of life. Become aware of how failure inevitably follows success, how happiness is transformed into varying degrees of unhappiness, how old age is inherent in youth, and how death is the natural consequence of life. Contemplate also that the converse of each of these is equally true. This is an extremely revealing practice, and it can be of great assistance in cultivating that nonattached posture which leads to real (unconditioned) happiness and real (unchanging) peace. Understanding the enslaving nature of duality (opposites, positive-negative) is the key to wisdom.

At the conclusion of this 5-minute period of contemplation, open your eyes and slowly extend your legs.

This terminates the meditation practice for today. (Make your notes.)

(Tomorrow's meditation practice requires a single flower of any variety, preferably contained in a small vase. Have these on hand for tomorrow's session.)

10th day
Flower

At this point in the course, it should be noted that beginning students are occasionally inclined to prejudge meditation practices. They will evaluate a particular technique as "difficult," "easy," "interesting," "boring," and so forth on the basis of how that technique strikes them at first glance. This is a serious error. Such students are as yet unaware that all seeds, regardless of their superficial appearance, have the identical objective: they serve as agents through which the mind and senses may be quieted and focused in the manner necessary to effect a transformation of consciousness. No beginning student can predict which of the meditation practices holds the key to his achievement of this one-pointed state. Unable to perceive the present condition of his consciousness, he cannot know to which of the seeds it will gravitate. Therefore, any judgment as to the degree of facility in the early stages of meditation is extremely unwise. With respect to this course, the student best serves himself by devoting his most serious efforts equally to each of the techniques presented. Only after he has completed the course will he be able to determine which, for him, is the most effective.

Today's practice, Flower Meditation, might be prejudged as "simple." It could appear that little more is involved than looking at a flower. Actually, as he absorbs the aspects of the flower, the student develops his ability in the "merging" technique, and he transforms his flower-gazing into a profound form of meditation. When he truly *sees* the flower, he knows that he has seen *all* things.

The student who has difficulty holding his attention on the seeds of other meditation practices frequently finds that the elements of the flower—design, color, texture—are those with which his mind can become more easily occupied. Once it is so engaged, meaningful concentration can follow.

Today's meditation requires a single flower of any variety. Place the flower, preferably contained in a small vase, in your meditation area before beginning today's Hatha Yoga routine.

Perform Hatha Yoga Elementary Routine A page 11

Open your eyes.

Place the flower in a position where you may comfortably fix your gaze on it. (Fig. 82.) Resume the cross-legged posture.

During the next 10 minutes, you are to become involved with the flower to the extent that none of the other senses and no thought will distract your attention. Visually examine its structure, form, texture, and color; attempt to discern the smallest detail of each. Take your time. Your concentration is total. If you perceive that your attention has wandered, that a sound or thought has distracted you, do not become impatient or reproach yourself; gently but firmly bring your mind back to the flower and continue your examination. As often as your mind wanders, return it to the flower. This is the only method for taming the mind and, eventually, bringing it under control.

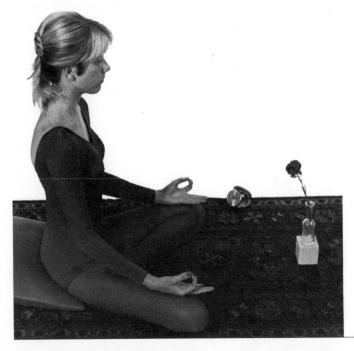

82. The meditator merges, effects Yoga, with the flower through total, unwavering, one-pointed focusing of the attention.

You will be able to *merge* with the flower to the extent that your concentration remains fixed. That is, if your mind and vision have been totally involved with the flower for several minutes without interruption, you begin to *become* the flower. You terminate the subject-object relationship. There is no longer a "you" who is looking at a flower; your identity is no longer separate from that of the flower. You *become* the flower and *effect* Yoga with it. You and the flower are ONE, and in this ONENESS there is no "you" and there is no "flower." There only IS.

Attempt to maintain this condition of ONENESS for the remainder of the session. Initially, you will probably be able to remain in this Yogic state for only a brief period. But even a few seconds will be a highly meaningful experience. Whenever this state of ONENESS dissolves during your practice, and the subject-object condition remanifests, attempt to merge again through the technique of total, unwavering concentration on the flower.

When the 10 minutes have elapsed, slowly extend your legs.

This terminates the meditation practice for today. (Make your notes.)

11th day

Alternate Nostril Breathing (2)

The value of Alternate Nostril Breathing for quieting the mind through balancing the positive-negative forces was described on the 5th Day. At that time, we performed this breathing technique in an elementary rhythm: 8-4-8. One of the most fascinating aspects of Alternate Nostril Breathing is that the depth of the quietude and awareness it produces can be gradually increased through modification of the counting rhythms. Each such modification presented in this course is slightly more advanced than that which precedes it and, as such, makes a greater demand on the breath-retention ability of the student. This ability is developed through continued practice, and the results are well worth the effort.

In today's performance of Alternate Nostril Breathing, the *retention* count alone is increased by 4 units, so that there is now a monomial rhythm of 8-8-8 for the inhalation, retention, and exhalation.

Perform Hatha Yoga Elementary Routine B page 23

83– Remain in the cross-legged posture with your left hand
84. in the *mudra*. Keep your eyes partially closed (only a slit of light should enter at the bottom).

Place the tip of your right thumb lightly against your right nostril and your ring and little fingers lightly against your left. Your index and middle fingers are together, and they rest lightly on your forehead (the "third eye" area).

Slowly and as quietly as possible, exhale deeply through both nostrils.

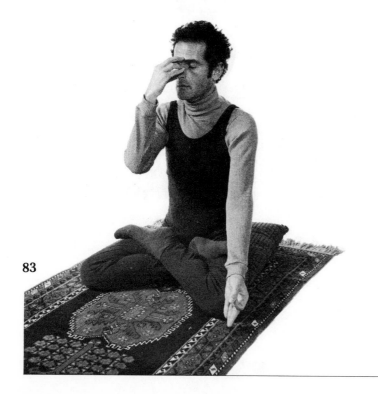

83

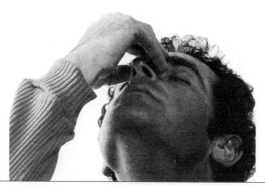

84

11th day

85. When the exhalation is completed, immediately close your right nostril by pressing your thumb against it. Slowly and quietly inhale deeply through your left nostril during a rhythmic count of 8.

86. Keep your right nostril closed and now press your left one so that both are closed. Retain the air for a rhythmic count of 8.

87. Release your right nostril (your left one remains closed) and exhale slowly, deeply, and quietly during a rhythmic count of 8.

88. When the air is completely exhaled, do not pause; immediately begin the next inhalation through your *right* nostril (the same nostril through which you just completed the exhalation). Inhale a deep, quiet breath through your right nostril during a rhythmic count of 8. Your left nostril remains closed.

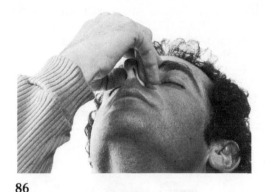

86

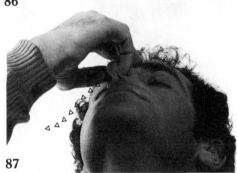

87

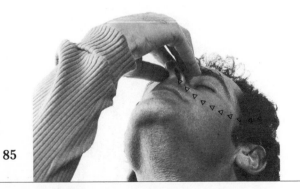

85

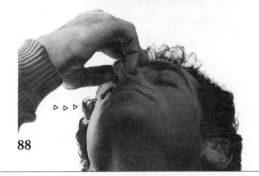

88

89. Keep your left nostril closed and now press your right one so that both are closed. Retain the air deep in your lungs during a rhythmic count of 8.

90. Release your left nostril (your right one remains closed) and exhale slowly, deeply, and quietly during a rhythmic count of 8.

You have now returned to the original starting point. Each time you return to this starting point, you have performed 1 complete round of Alternate Nostril Breathing.

Without pause, keep your right nostril closed and begin the next round with a deep, quiet inhalation through your left nostril during a rhythmic count of 8.

Perform 7 rounds.

Lower your right hand and place it (in the *mudra*) on your right knee (or thigh). (Fig. 91.)

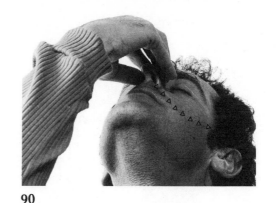

90

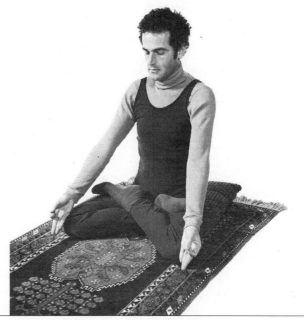

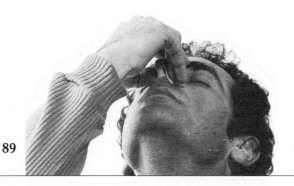

89

91

11th day

Summary

inhale through left	count 8
retain; both closed	count 8
exhale through right	count 8

without pause

inhale through right	count 8
retain; both closed	count 8
exhale through left	count 8

This completes 1 round. Without pause, begin the next round.

Do not permit your breath to gush or hiss in or out. Perform the inhalations and exhalations as quietly as possible. Think of the breathing as occurring more in the throat than the nostrils.

The counting is rhythmic and continuous, it is never interrupted. Once the counting begins, you keep it going like a metronome, steady and rhythmic.

Throughout the exercise, your attention must be fully focused on the counting. It must not become automatic while your attention is allowed to wander. Total concentration on the counting, in conjunction with respiration, is the seed for this meditation practice.

When you have completed the 7 rounds, remain seated quietly for a short interval, and you will become aware of the profound state of quietude that has resulted from your practice. Note particularly the extent to which your breathing has been slowed. This illustrates that when the mind is quiet, the breathing is slow and regular. Conversely, when you practice to make your breathing slow and regular, your mind can become steady and one-pointed. (Fig. 91.)

Open your eyes and slowly extend your legs.

This terminates the meditation practice for today. (Make your notes.)

12th day
Yantra (3)

The triangle is a symbol universally employed in mystical practices and sacred structures. The extraordinary properties of the pyramidal form, consisting of a series of triangles, are currently receiving more attention in the Western world than ever before. For students of meditation, the esoteric value of the triangle lies in its *integrating* quality. Ordinarily, the diverse aspects of one's existence—the physical, emotional, and mental bodies—pull against and contend with one another for attention and gratification. Experiencing this continual internal warfare, the ordinary person finds himself restless, insecure, always seeking new ways in which to realize a sense of fulfillment. As quickly as he quenches the thirst of one body, new demands for gratification arise from the others. The visualization of the triangle is one of the methods we use for unifying the physical, emotional, and mental bodies so that they function as an integrated unit. With this integration accomplished, the turmoil diminishes and large amounts of energy that were formerly consumed in the conflict can now be directed into achieving greater efficiency in everyday activities as well as more productive Yoga practice.

In this book, we are not concerned with how and why the visualization of the yantras—or the practice of any of our meditation techniques—accomplishes the indicated objectives. In the context of this 30 Day course, such involved explanations simply serve to cater to the intellect—the ordinary mind. It is this very intellect which is obscuring our true nature, our ONENESS; it is this ordinary mind which we are working to transcend. To know that the techniques *do* accomplish their purposes is sufficient at this time. They are tried and proven. Nonetheless, it is you who will ultimately evaluate their effectiveness by the results you experience through serious, patient, and regular practice.

Today, we will visualize the triangle first in its fundamental form and then encompassed by a circle. (It is not a coincidence that the Lotus postures place the body into a triangular form. Each time you assume a cross-legged position, you are proclaiming your integration as well as accumulating additional energy that enters through the crown of the head, the apex of the triangle.)

Perform Hatha Yoga Elementary Routine C page 31

Remain in the cross-legged posture. Open your eyes.

Place the book in a position where you may comfortably fix your gaze on Fig. 93. Both your gaze and attention must remain fully fixed on the figure. (Fig. 92.)*

Direct your eyes slowly from the apex of the triangle to the bottom of the right side, across the base from right to

*If you had to come out of the cross-legged posture to properly position the book, resume the posture before beginning meditation practice.

left, and then up the left side to the apex. Repeat this procedure for 2 minutes.

Now close your eyes and visualize the identical figure for 3 minutes. Do not allow your attention to wander; no thoughts should enter your mind. If the image begins to fade, or if you perceive that your attention has wandered, remanifest the figure by constructing it in the clockwise direction described above.

When the 3 minutes have elapsed, open your eyes.

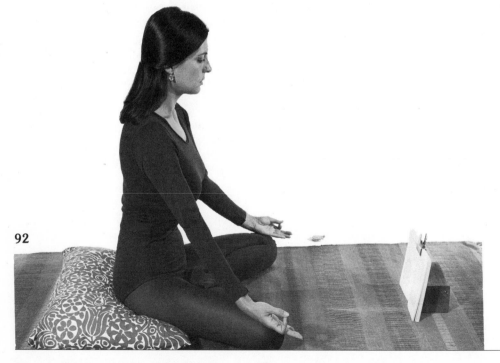

92

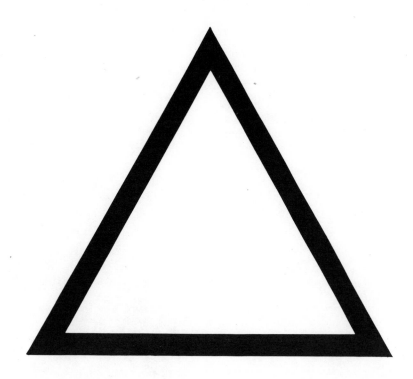

93. Yantra 3: the equilateral triangle.

12th day

Fix your gaze on Fig. 95. You will note that the triangle is now encompassed by a circle. Hold your gaze steadily on this figure for 2 minutes.

When the 2 minutes have elapsed, close your eyes and visualize the identical figure for 3 minutes. If the image fades, remanifest it by constructing a clockwise triangle and then enclosing it with a clockwise circle. (All yantras may be visualized in black, white, or color.)

If you are still finding the visualizations weak, reinforce the image by opening your eyes and observing the figure on the page for a few additional moments. Then close your eyes and make another attempt.

When the 3 minutes have elapsed, open your eyes and slowly extend your legs.

This terminates the meditation practice for today. (Make your notes.)

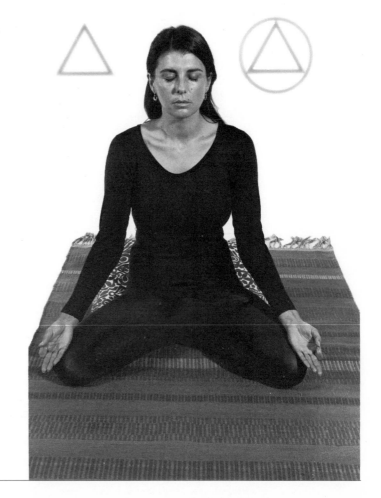

94. The simple (left) and more complex yantras are visualized successively.

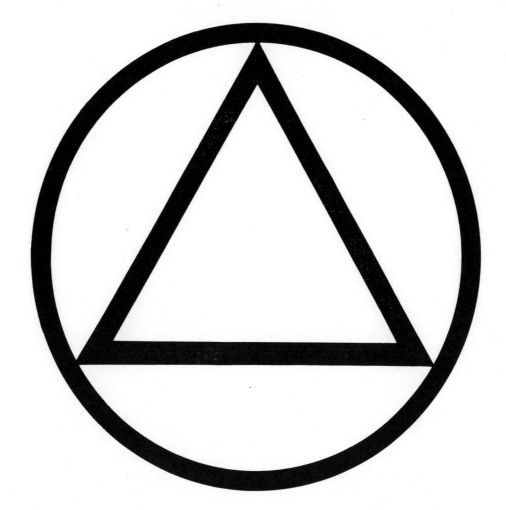

95. The fundamental yantra encompassed by a circle.

Hatha Yoga

INTERMEDIATE ROUTINE A

For Use on Days 13, 16, 19

According to your ability, you may
either perform these intermediate
positions or remain with the elementary
positions and work toward the gradual
accomplishment of this more advanced
practice. Your body will advise you of
the best procedure in each *asana*.
You must never strain or experience
persistent discomfort in Hatha Yoga.

It may be that you are able to perform
the intermediate positions of some *asanas*
but still only the elementary positions
of others. This is perfectly satisfactory.
Simply continue to work toward the
gradual accomplishment of the
intermediate position of each *asana*.

Remember that you begin each
asana in the starting position
learned in the Elementary Routines.

chest expansion

96. The upright position.

97. The backward bend position (a moderate increase from the elementary position). Arms are held away from back, knees remain straight, and eyes look upward. Hold motionless for 5.

98. The forward bend (an increase of several inches from the elementary position). Bring arms into position indicated. Knees are straight and neck is limp. Hold motionless for 10.

Slowly straighten to upright position and repeat once.

Unclasp hands and gracefully lower yourself into seated position.

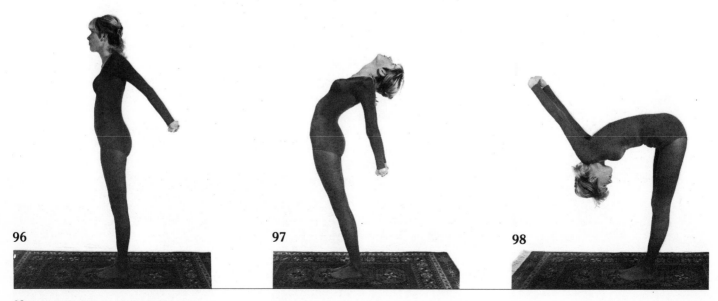

96   97   98

knee-and-thigh stretch

99. The beginning position.

100. You may now be able to lower knees an increased distance toward floor. Hold trunk erect and maintain stretch for a count of 10. Relax hands and arms for a few moments. During this relaxation, knees can be raised. Repeat. Perform 3 times.

Unclasp hands. Move gracefully into a lying position. Stomach and forehead rest on mat.

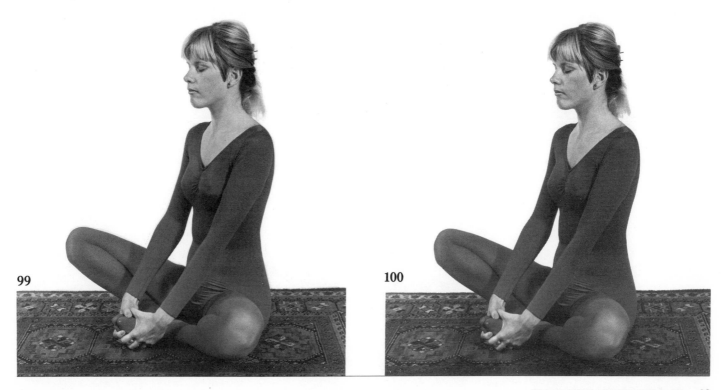

99

100

cobra

101. The elementary raised position.

102. Trunk is raised to intermediate position.
The raise is executed in very slow motion; head
is always back and spine continually curved.
Hold without motion for 10. Legs are relaxed.

In very slow motion, reverse the movements and
lower trunk until forehead once again rests on mat.

Relax a few moments and repeat. Perform 3 times.
Relax with forehead on mat.

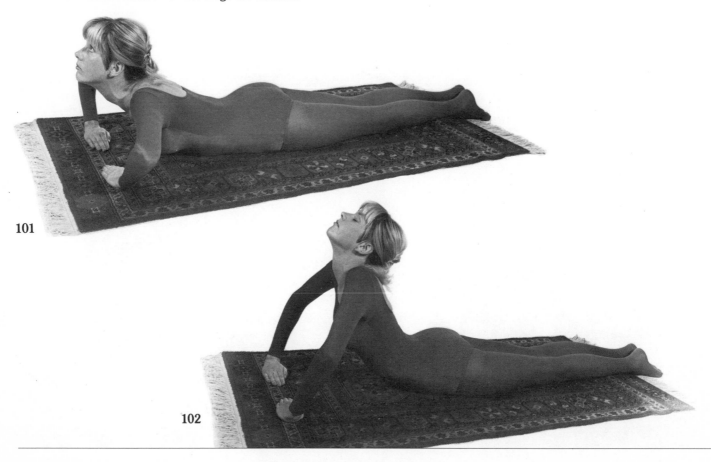

101

102

head twist

103–
104.
Technically, there are no intermediate positions for the Head Twist. The movements are identical with those you performed in the elementary routine. However, it is possible that as you continue to practice these movements, your neck will loosen and your head can be moved slightly farther in each of the three directions.

Perform the movements as previously, holding the extreme position of each for a count of 20. Do the routine twice.

Rest chin on mat and lower arms to sides.

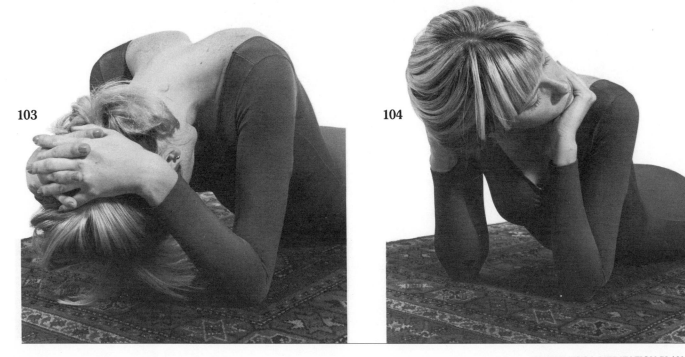

103

104

bow

105. The beginning position.

106. The distance of the raise is increased from that of the elementary routine to approximately the position illustrated. Head is held high and knees are as close together as possible. Breathe normally. Hold without motion for 10.

Lower knees and chin to floor, but retain the hold on feet. Pause a few moments and repeat. Perform 3 times. Following final repetition, release feet and lower them slowly to floor. Rest cheek on mat and relax.

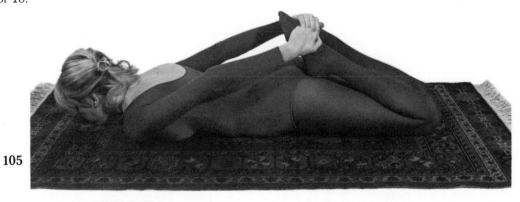

105

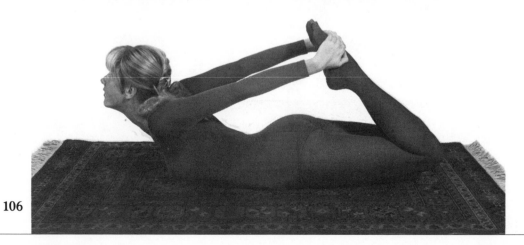

106

Observation of the Breath

Sit in cross-legged posture and observe the breath for 1 minute as instructed on page 21.

Hatha Yoga

INTERMEDIATE ROUTINE B

For Use on Days 14, 17, 20

All starting positions are identical with those learned in Elementary Routine B.

rishi's posture

107. Trunk and arms turned left to the 90-degree position.

108. Right hand takes a firm hold on back of right calf while gaze follows left hand to position illustrated. Hold without motion for 10.

Slowly raise trunk, bring extended arms into frontward position. Twist slowly to right and perform the identical movements. Perform 3 times to each side, alternating left-right.

Following final repetition, slowly lower arms to sides and relax.

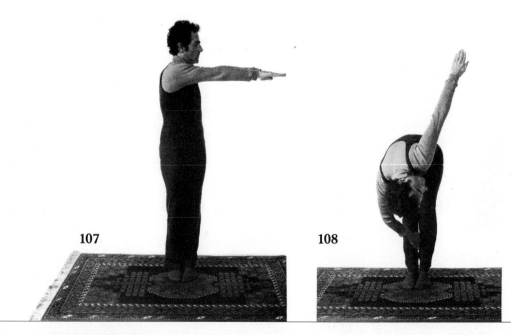

107   108

balance posture

109. The beginning position.

110. Left arm moves slightly backward, eyes look directly upward, and right foot is pulled gently upward as high as possible.
Hold with as little motion as possible for 5.

Slowly return foot to floor and arms to sides.

Perform the identical movements on opposite side.

Perform 3 times on each side, alternating sides.

Following final repetition, lower yourself gracefully into a seated position on mat.

(Total balance may be slow in developing. Do not be discouraged. Continued practice will bring success.)

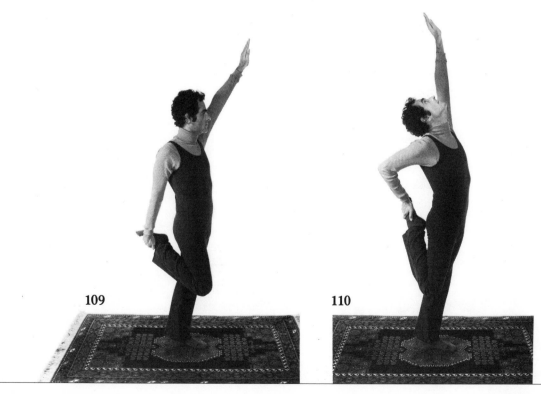

109

110

alternate leg stretch

111. In the beginning position, trunk bends backward several inches. Head is back and eyes look upward.

112. During slow-motion forward dive, trunk comes forward a sufficient distance so that both hands may take a firm hold on left ankle. Pull against ankle and slowly lower trunk as far as possible without strain. Elbows bend slightly outward and forehead is aimed at knee. Hold without motion for 10.

Slowly straighten trunk to upright position.

Raise arms slowly and repeat the movements. Perform 3 times.

Perform the identical movements 3 times with right leg extended. Following final repetition, extend left leg and rest hands on thighs.

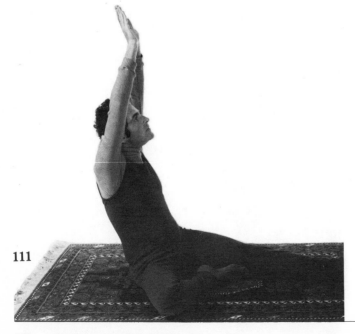

111

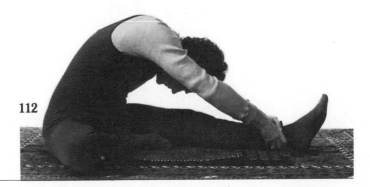

112

backward bend

113. The starting position. Knees must remain together throughout the movements.

114. Inch backward as far as possible. Arms remain parallel with sides, fingers are together and point directly away from back. Slowly arch trunk upward as far as possible and lower head backward as far as possible. Remain seated on heels. Hold without motion for 10.

Raise head, relax trunk, and rest a few moments, but maintain position of arms.

Once again, slowly arch trunk upward and lower head backward. Remain seated on heels. Hold for 10.

Raise head, lower trunk, and slowly move hands and trunk forward to starting position of Fig. 113.

Come off heels, swing legs around, and extend them straight outward.

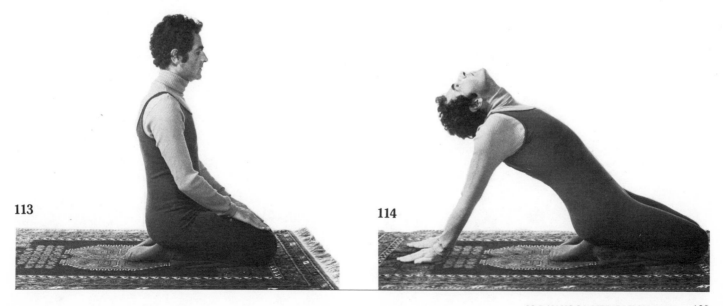

113

114

twist

115. Legs are extended.

Bend right knee and position right leg as illustrated.

Cross left leg over right leg and position it as illustrated. Sole of left foot is on floor, close to right knee.

Place left hand firmly on floor behind back.

Cross right arm over left knee and hold right knee.

116. Very slowly twist trunk and head a moderate distance to left. Hold without motion for 10.

Maintain position of hands, but slowly turn trunk frontward so that you return to position of Fig. 115.

Relax a few moments. Repeat twisting of trunk. Perform 3 twists.

Following final repetition, turn frontward, extend both legs.

Perform the identical movements on right side by exchanging the words "left" and "right" in the above directions. Perform 3 times to right side.

Following final repetition, turn frontward, extend both legs, and assume cross-legged posture.

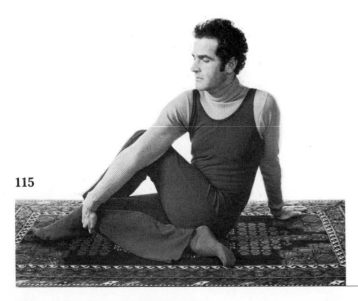

115

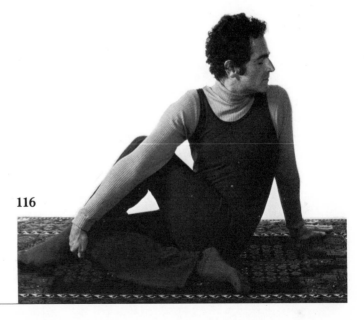

116

Observation of the Breath

Sit in cross-legged posture and observe the breath for 1 minute as instructed on page 21.

Hatha Yoga

INTERMEDIATE ROUTINE C

For Use on Days 15, 18, 21

All starting positions are identical with those learned in Elementary Routine C.

triangle

117. Assume an intermediate stance and gracefully raise arms to shoulder level.

118. Slowly bend to left and hold left calf.

Pull on calf and lower trunk to approximately the position illustrated. Bring right arm (with elbow straight) over head to position illustrated. Allow neck to relax. Hold for 10.

Slowly straighten to upright position of Fig. 117.

Execute the identical movements to right. Perform 3 times to each side, alternating left-right.

Following final repetition, bring arms to sides, gracefully draw legs together, and lower yourself into a seated position on mat.

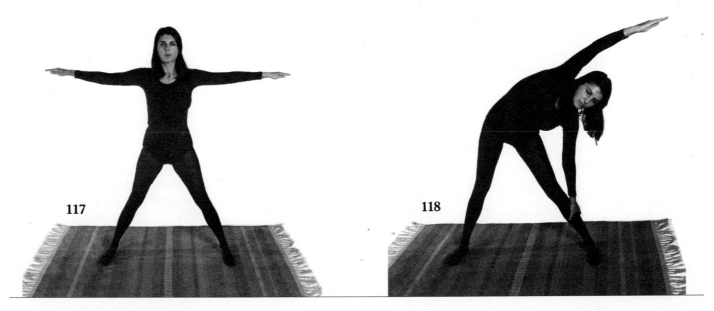

117

118

back stretch

119. Extend both legs straight outward.

In very slow motion, raise arms to overhead position and bend backward several inches to position illustrated. Look upward.

120. During slow-motion forward dive, trunk comes forward a sufficient distance so that hands may firmly hold ankles. Pull against ankles and slowly lower trunk as far as possible without strain. Elbows bend slightly outward and forehead is aimed at knees. Hold without motion for 10.

Slowly straighten trunk to upright position.

Raise arms slowly and repeat the movements. Perform 3 times.

Following final repetition, straighten trunk to upright position, rest hands on thighs, and slowly lower back to floor.

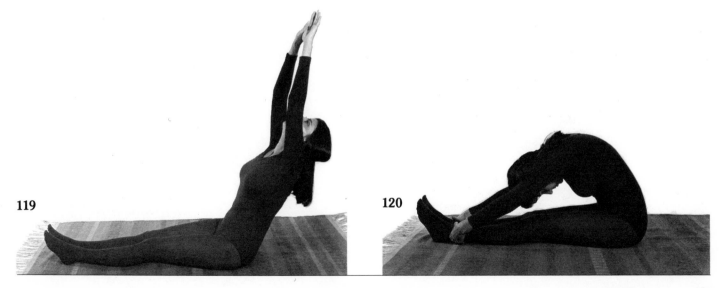

119

120

shoulder stand

121. Bring legs back gracefully over head.

122. Brace hands against hips and raise trunk and legs to
intermediate position illustrated. Relax body and
breathe normally. Hold for 1–2 minutes.

Slowly lower legs behind head for the Plough *asana*.

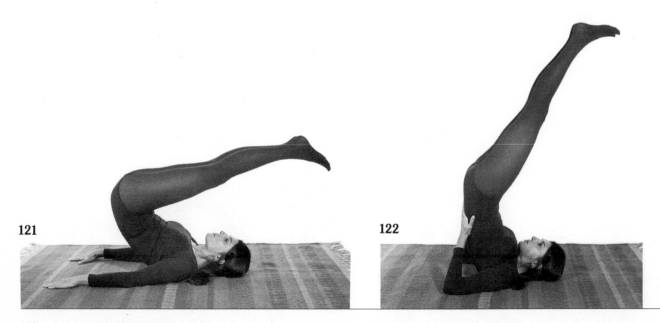

121

122

plough

123. From the Shoulder Stand position, slowly lower legs toward floor. Knees are straight. Brace palms against floor.

124. Touch toes to floor, hold knees straight. Chin is pressed tightly against upper chest. Control breathing so that it is slow and rhythmic. Hold without motion for 1 minute.

The procedure for coming out of the position is identical with that of the elementary routine.

Relax a few moments in prone position and then come into seated cross-legged posture.

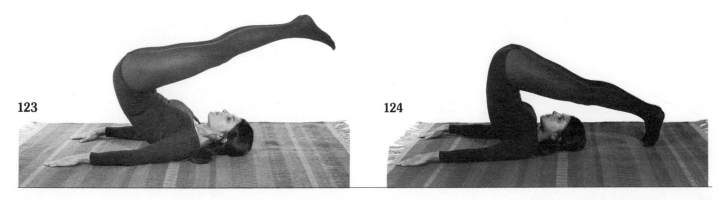

123

124

head roll

125– Technically, there are no intermediate positions for
126. the Head Roll. The movements are identical with
those you performed in the elementary routine.
However, it is possible that as you continue to practice these movements, your neck will loosen and
your head can be moved slightly farther in each of
the four positions. Perform the movements as previously, holding the extreme position of each for a
count of 10. Do the routine twice.

Upon completion, remain in cross-legged posture,
keep eyes closed, and raise head.

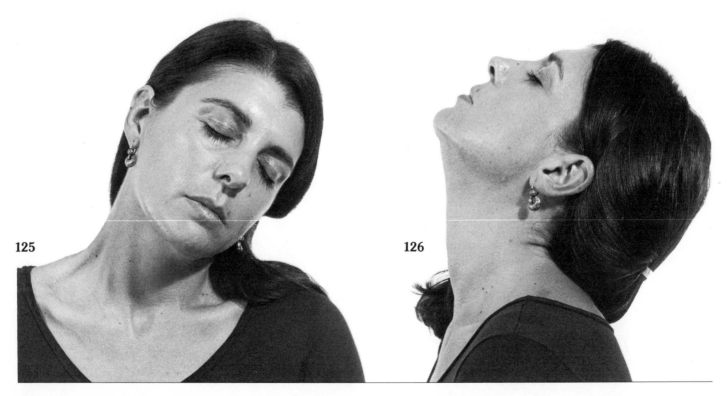

125

126

Observation of the Breath

   Sit in cross-legged posture and observe the breath for 1
minute as instructed on page 21.

13th day

OM (2)

Through lengthening the intonation of the sounds of OM, we increase the mantra's effectiveness. On the 6th Day, the counting rhythm for the syllables was 2-2-4. Today, that rhythm is doubled. The silent segment—which is comprised of completion of the exhalation and the inhalation that follows—is the same as previously. The student must now be aware that this silence is the *withdrawal* aspect of the cosmological cycle. The complete cycle is, then, A = the creation, U = the preservation, M = the dissolution, and silence = the withdrawal period of the universe when it is unmanifest and reposes in its *potential* state. Therefore, the intoning of the supreme mantra, OM, places the meditator in concord with the eternal cycle and, consequently, with the ONE through which the cycle moves. This concordance is Yoga. ("... the Word was with God, and the Word *was* God.")

Perform Hatha Yoga Intermediate Routine A page 91

Remain in the cross-legged posture. Your eyelids are partially lowered.

Exhale deeply.

In a count of 4 (approximating seconds), inhale deeply and quietly.

In a firm, steady, controlled voice, produce the sound "Oh" from the back of your mouth. (Fig. 127.) This should be performed in a count of 4.

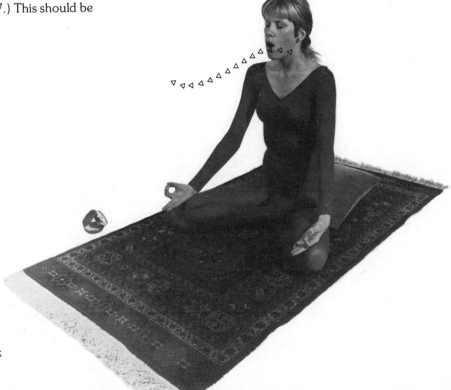

127. The "Oh" sound proceeds from back of mouth; lips in "o" shape.

13th day

Without interruption, continue the "Oh" sound, but now let it proceed from the front of your mouth. As it moves to the front, it assumes a slightly nasal quality. (Fig. 128.) This second sound is also performed in a count of 4.

Without interruption, press your lips together and produce the sound "Mmmm." (Fig. 129.) This sound should resonate strongly, like the buzzing of a bee, and you should feel the vibrations throughout your head and chest. Perform this in a count of 8.

Keep your lips together and *silently* complete the exhalation so that your lungs are emptied during an additional count of 2.

Without interruption, inhale deeply and quietly in a count of 4. (The completion of the exhalation and inhalation represents the silence and withdrawal that follows dissolution and precedes creation.)

Repeat the mantra. Devote 5 minutes to *japa* (repetition). You will be able to perform approximately 13 repetitions during this period. (See Summary page 116.)

When the 5 minutes have elapsed, sit very quietly for another 5 minutes and become aware of what is transpiring within. Focus your attention fully on what you are experiencing and do not allow your mind to wander.

When the 5 minutes have elapsed, open your eyes and slowly extend your legs.

This terminates the meditation practice for today. (Make your notes.)

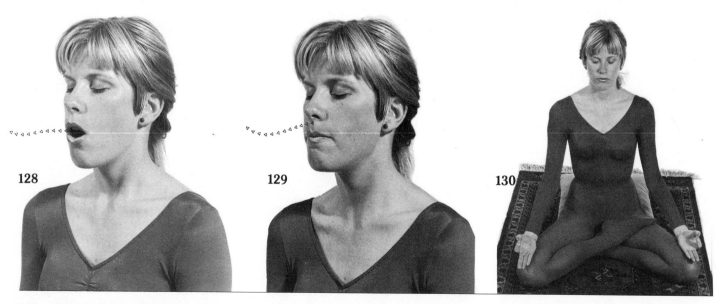

128   129   130

Summary

	Deep inhalation	"Oh"	"Oh"	"Mmmm"	Finish exhalation
Sound characteristics	Silent	Proceeds from back of mouth; lips in "o" shape	Transferred to front of mouth; has slight nasal quality; lips remain in "o" shape	Lips together; strong resonance vibrating throughout head and chest	Silent
Time (attempt to approximate seconds)	4	4	4	8	2

The rhythm remains steady: an uninterrupted 4, 4-4-8, 2.
Fix this rhythm firmly in your mind before beginning the practice.

The voice is steady, firm, controlled, and remains on the same pitch.

The attention is fully focused on the sound. You must not allow the *japa* to become automatic while your mind and senses wander.

128. "Oh" sound is transferred to front of mouth and has slight nasal quality; lips remain in "o" shape.

129. Lips together; strong vibrations of "Mmmm" throughout head and chest.

130. The attention is fixed on what is transpiring within.

14th day

Asana Meditation (2)

You are now sufficiently familiar with the *asanas* of Routine B to utilize them as seeds for meditation. The technique is identical with that which we applied to Routine A on the 7th Day. The *asana* is converted from a physical exercise to a meditation practice by totally immersing the mind in the *feeling* of the movements and by becoming aware of their effects on the areas of the body that are involved. Additionally, during the hold segment of the *asana,* the attention is directed to that area of the body where the maximum emphasis is experienced.

This technique focuses the mind in the one-pointed manner and, through intense concentration, accelerates progress in the *asanas.* The student begins to understand that ultimately Hatha Yoga is a discipline more for the mind than for the body! Learning to become aware of what transpires within the body as a result of *asana* practice is the prelude to transcending the self through Hatha Yoga.

Perform Hatha Yoga Intermediate Routine B page 99

Repeat the identical routine of Hatha Yoga *asanas* that you performed today. The posture will now be performed *with your total attention focused on all of the movements.* You are to *feel* their effects on the areas of the body that are involved.

The arrows indicate those particular areas of the body which receive the greatest emphasis during the hold. Direct your consciousness to the indicated area and maintain it there for the duration of the hold. If you detect that your attention is wandering, return it immediately to the movements or the hold.

Rest briefly between *asanas*. The number of repetitions for the *asanas* in this meditation routine differs from that of the regular routine.

Now stand up gracefully, turn your attention inward, and perform the routine.

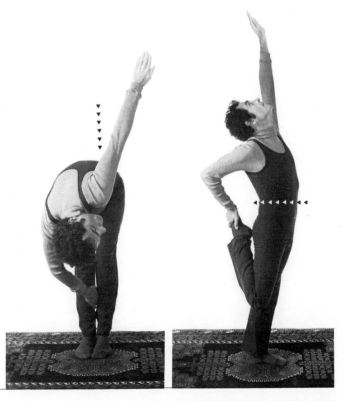

131. Hold for 10 on each side. Perform twice to each side, alternating left-right.

132. Hold for 5 on each side. Perform twice on each side, alternating sides.

14th day

133. Hold for 20 with each leg. Perform twice with left leg and then twice with right leg.

134. Hold for 10. Perform stretching position twice. (Remain seated on heels between repetitions.)

135. Hold for 20 on each side. Perform twice to the left side and then twice to the right side. During each hold, your consciousness is directed to the spiral formation of your lower and middle spine.

Upon completion of the routine, assume the cross-legged posture and rest for approximately 1 minute with your eyes partially closed. Become aware of how your body feels at this point.

Open your eyes and slowly extend your legs.

This terminates the meditation practice for today. (Make your notes.)

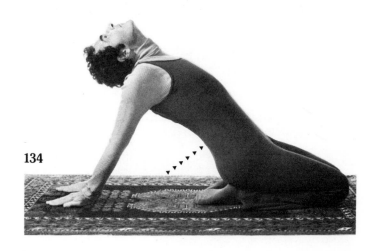

134

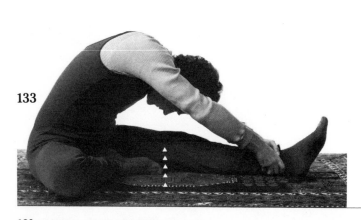

133

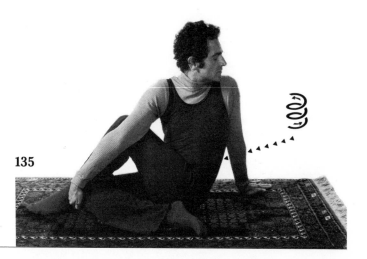

135

15th day

Deep Relaxation: A Path to the Void

Today marks the halfway point in our *30 Day Plan.*

For the past 14 days, we have used various seeds for the meditation sessions; we have occupied the body, mind, and senses by presenting them with something—an object, a mantra, a posture—upon which to focus. A major objective of this focusing is to gain aptitude in concentration, in achieving the essential one-pointed state. Now that some ability has been developed for this objective, we want to begin to experience what occurs *when there is no seed*—no object, no thing—to which the consciousness is directed. We attempt to locate the "off" button and, by pushing it, temporarily eliminate all thoughts and sensations.

The student may be inclined to prejudge this as a practice which renders the mind blank and results in nothingness. We are accustomed to think of "nothing" as the opposite of "something." But the void that is experienced through meditation is anything but empty. The student grows to recognize that what was conceived of as nothingness contains the greatest fullness, and that the essence of this fullness—from which all things emanate—can be perceived only when no thoughts and emotions are superimposed upon it. Thoughts, and the emotions that accompany them, distract and prevent one from Knowing his true nature as that of the Void; all things exist within him, and he exists in all things. When the beginning meditator transcends the self and merges with the Void (achieves Yoga), if only for a few moments, it is as though he were in the eye of the hurricane: he may still sense that the phantoms of turbulence surround him, but he is at peace in his total quietude. Gradually, he learns how to extend this quietude from the meditation session to his daily activities.

In our previous performance of Deep Relaxation (1st Day), we practiced to gain the *feeling* of the body in the totally relaxed state. Today, we again place the body in this relaxed condition, but now, rather than focusing on the feeling of this state, we allow the consciousness to transcend all phenomena—all thoughts, visions, and sensations—and to merge with the All-In-All of the Void. Classically, this practice is known as "meditation without seed."

Perform Hatha Yoga Intermediate Routine C page 107

From the cross-legged posture, slowly extend your legs straight outward.

Slowly lower your back to the floor.

Place your arms as illustrated in Fig. 136. Palms face upward. Close your eyes. Breathe normally.

Allow your body to become limp.

The procedure is identical with that of the 1st Day. Beginning with your feet, direct your consciousness very slowly and very deliberately through your body, relaxing each area in turn: feet, calves, thighs, buttocks, groin, abdomen, chest, back; then down to your hands and up through your arms, shoulders, neck, jaw, and face. (If you have any doubts regarding this procedure, do not hesitate to refer to the instructions of the 1st Day.)

Remain in the relaxed condition for several moments and observe your breathing.

Now, to be certain that you have allowed each set of

muscles to let go completely so that the ultimate state of relaxation is attained, repeat the exercise. Therefore, once again, very slowly and deliberately direct your consciousness through your entire body, becoming sensitive to all areas that may have remained tensed, however slightly.

When your attention has moved into your facial area for the second time, approximately 5 minutes will have elapsed, and your body should be in the totally relaxed state.

Now let go of all feelings and thoughts. The mind is turned off. Dismiss any thought, vision, or sensation that arises. Do not direct your consciousness; allow it to sink as it will. Remain acutely aware of whatever transpires; do not associate this state with that of sleep.

Maintain total quietude for approximately 5 minutes. When this period has elapsed, open your eyes, slowly raise your trunk and come into a seated position.

This terminates the meditation practice for today. (Make your notes.)

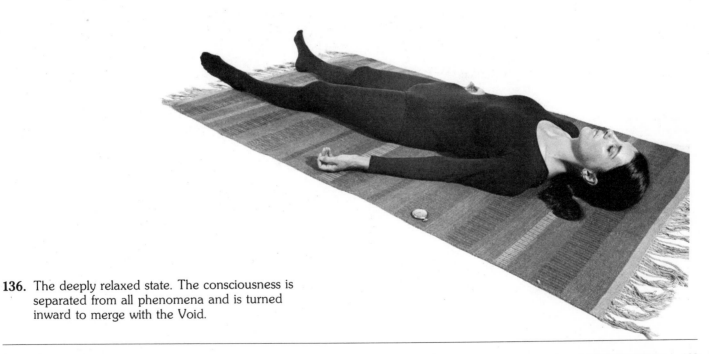

136. The deeply relaxed state. The consciousness is separated from all phenomena and is turned inward to merge with the Void.

16th day

Yantra (4)

Today's yantra is symbolic of the *ascension of consciousness.* *

The meditator's objective is to elevate and thereby transform his consciousness. Although the serious student intellectually understands the value of being constantly aware of his objective, this awareness frequently slips away amidst the course of daily activities because the consciousness, operating on the gross level through the mind and senses, is hypnotized, lulled to sleep by these activities. As curious as it may seem, the fact is that the student needs to be frequently awakened and reminded of his objective! Therefore, techniques to effect awakening and Self-remembering must be regularly introduced into his practice. The visualization of the ascending spiral is one such technique. It not only serves as a reminder, but assists in reinforcing the student's resolve to elevate and refine his consciousness in that degree necessary for it to merge with its source (Yoga). The spiral yantra impresses a pattern of ascension upon the consciousness and it responds accordingly.

*In that form of Yoga known as *Laya,* the ascension of consciousness is inherent in the activation of the *kundalini* force.

Instructions

Perform Hatha Yoga Intermediate Routine A page 91

Remain in the cross-legged posture. Open your eyes.

Place the book in a position where you may comfortably fix your gaze on Fig. 138. Both your gaze and attention must remain fully fixed on the figure. (Fig. 137.)*

Direct your eyes slowly from the bottom of the spiral, along the ascending lines, to the top. When you reach top, drop your eyes *directly* down to the bottom.

Repeat this procedure for 5 minutes. (Today's practice is divided into two 5-minute segments. Previously, the yantra segments were limited to 2 and 3 minutes.)

Now close your eyes and visualize the identical figure for the second 5-minute period. Do not allow your attention to wander; no thoughts should enter your mind. If the image begins to fade, or if you perceive that your attention has wandered, remanifest the figure by constructing it in the ascending fashion. (All yantras may be visualized in black, white or color.)

*If you had to come out of the cross-legged posture to properly position the book, resume the posture before beginning meditation practice.

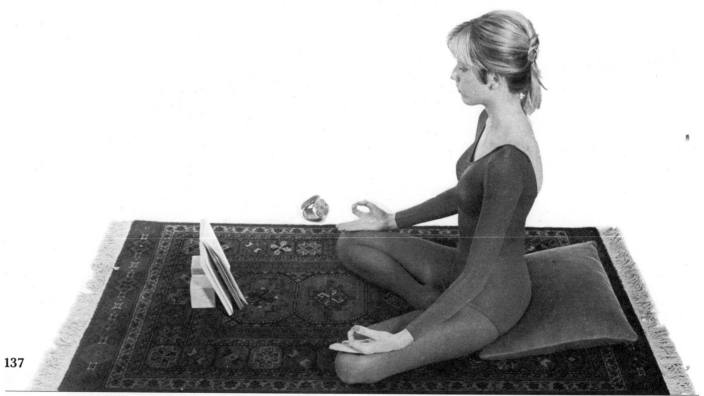

137

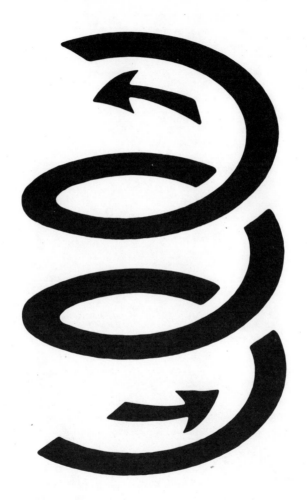

138. Yantra 4: the ascending spiral.

16th day

If you find the visualization weak, reinforce the image by opening your eyes and observing the figure on the page for a few additional moments. Then close your eyes and make another attempt.

When the 5 minutes have elapsed, open your eyes and slowly extend your legs.

This terminates the meditation practice for today. (Make your notes.)

(Tomorrow's meditation requires incense. Any incense that is pleasing to you is satisfactory. Have the incense and its holder on hand for tomorrow's session.)

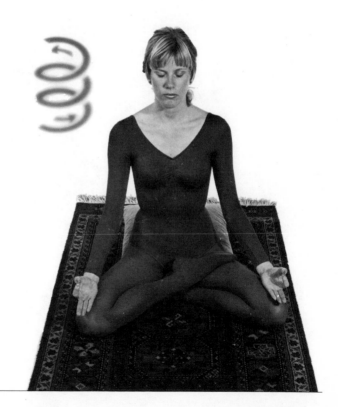

139. The yantra is visualized for 5 minutes.

17th day

Incense

In our 30 Day course, certain of the senses, occupied with suggested objects, are utilized as seeds for meditation. As each of these senses becomes a seed, it assumes the completely dominant position; the student practices to have his consciousness totally involved with *that* sense, the other senses being temporarily in limbo or de-sensitized. In today's meditation, the olfactory sense, occupied with incense, is the seed.

For countless centuries, incense has been used in places of worship throughout the world. Its function in this context is twofold: first, it serves, together with other accoutrements, to create an atmosphere, an environment for the appropriate rituals; second, the adherent grows to associate the scent of a particular incense with the place of worship where it is used and with all that transpires there. Consequently, any encounter with that odor—upon entering the temple, at home, or elsewhere—can be expected to produce the same spiritually receptive state that has been previously experienced.

People respond differently to different types of incense. For some, a certain scent may have properties that will actually change their moods and even alter their state of consciousness. For others, the same scent produces no such effects. This is unimportant here. Our concern is with achieving the one-pointed state, and the value of the incense for us is that it provides an effective seed for concentration. The olfactory sense is quickly captivated, and the attention can be easily drawn to and held by the incense. For many beginning students, Incense Meditation is the best technique for merging with the seed and experiencing the state of ONENESS (Yoga).

Today's meditation requires lighted incense. Any incense that is pleasing to you will be satisfactory. Place the incense (in its holder) and a match in your meditation area before beginning today's Hatha Yoga routine.

Perform Hatha Yoga Intermediate Routine B page 99

Open your eyes.

Light the incense and place it approximately 2 feet from where you will be seated (Fig. 140.) You must be able to detect the scent with ease, but it must not be overpowering. If necessary, adjust the distance during meditation.

Seated in the cross-legged posture, lower your eyelids, but do not close your eyes entirely.

During the next 10 minutes, fix your attention on the incense and do not permit it to be distracted. Become totally involved with the scent. Determine if it is heavy, light, strong, subtle, sweet, and the like. Take your time in noting these various qualities. If you perceive that your attention has wandered, return it to the scent and resume your examination.

You will be able to *merge* with the scent to the extent that your concentration remains fixed. That is, if your mind and sense of smell have been totally involved with the incense for several minutes without interruption, you begin to *become* the scent. You terminate the subject-object relationship. There is no longer a "you" who is smelling the incense; your identity is no longer separate from that of the scent. You *become* the scent and effect Yoga with it. You and the scent are ONE, and in this ONENESS there is no "you" and there is no "scent." There only IS.

Attempt to maintain this condition of ONENESS for the remainder of the session. Whenever this state dissolves during your practice, and the subject-object condition remanifests, attempt to merge again through the technique of total, unwavering concentration on the scent.

When the 10 minutes have elapsed, slowly extend your legs.

This terminates the meditation practice for today. (Make your notes.)

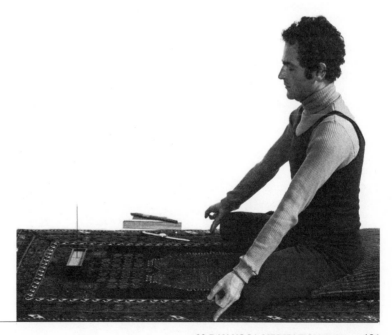

140. The meditator merges, effects Yoga, with the scent of the incense through total, unwavering, one-pointed focusing of the attention.

18th day
Alternate Nostril Breathing (3)

In today's practice of this technique, the counting rhythm for the three segments is again modified. Whereas on the 11th Day the inhalation, retention, and exhalation were performed in the monomial rhythm of 8-8-8, now the inhalation is decreased to 4, the retention is increased to 16, and the exhalation remains at 8. This ratio of 1:4:2 further increases the effectiveness of Alternate Nostril Breathing in promoting the positive-negative balance of *prana*.

Following your performance of 7 rounds in today's rhythm, you should have a definite sense of that profound quietude in which the mind is stilled, the consciousness elevated, and the ego temporarily transcended.

Instructions

Perform Hatha Yoga Intermediate Routine C page 107

141 – Remain in the cross-legged posture with your left hand
142. in the *mudra*. Keep your eyes partially closed (only a slit of light should enter at the bottom).

Place the tip of your right thumb lightly against your right nostril and your ring and little fingers lightly against your left. Your index and middle fingers are together, and they rest lightly on your forehead (the "third eye" area).

Slowly and as quietly as possible, exhale deeply through both nostrils.

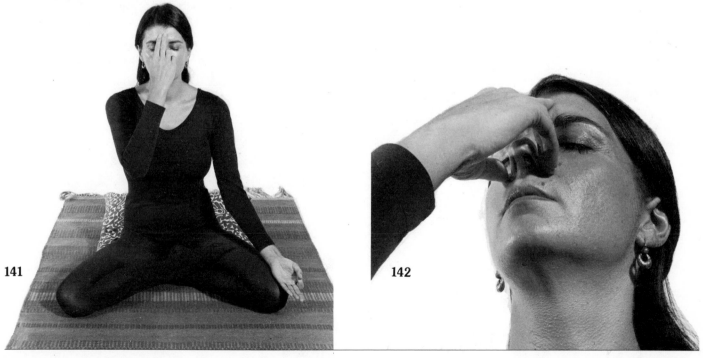

141

142

18th day

143. When the exhalation is completed, immediately close your right nostril by pressing your thumb against it. Slowly and quietly inhale deeply through your left nostril during a rhythmic count of 4.

144. Keep your right nostril closed and now press your left one so that both are closed. Retain the air for a rhythmic count of 16.

145. Release your right nostril (your left one remains closed) and exhale slowly, deeply, and quietly during a rhythmic count of 8.

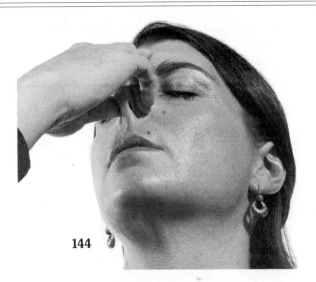

144

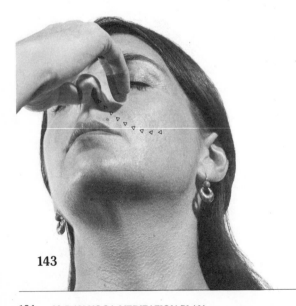

143

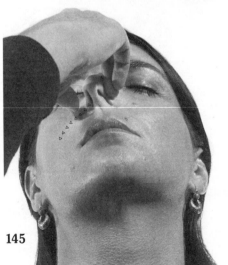

145

146. When the air is completely exhaled, do not pause; immediately begin the next inhalation through your *right* nostril (the same nostril through which you just completed the exhalation). Inhale a deep, quiet breath through your right nostril during a rhythmic count of 4. Your left nostril remains closed.

147. Keep your left nostril closed and now press your right one so that both are closed. Retain the air deep in your lungs during a rhythmic count of 16.

148. Release your left nostril (your right one remains closed) and exhale slowly, deeply, and quietly during a rhythmic count of 8.

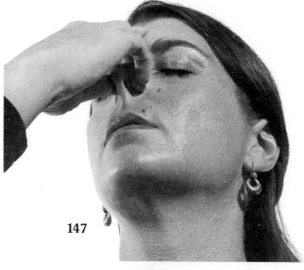

147

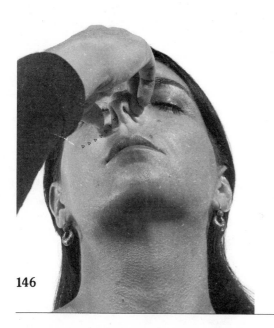

146

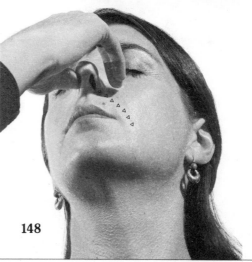

148

18th day

You have now returned to the original starting point. Each time you return to this starting point, you have performed 1 complete round of Alternate Nostril Breathing.

Without pause, keep your right nostril closed and begin the next round with a deep, quiet inhalation through your left nostril during a rhythmic count of 4. Perform 7 rounds.

149. Lower your right hand and place it (in the *mudra*) on your right knee (or thigh).

Summary

inhale through left	count 4
retain; both closed	count 16
exhale through right	count 8
without pause	
inhale through right	count 4
retain; both closed	count 16
exhale through left	count 8

This completes 1 round. Without pause, begin the next round.

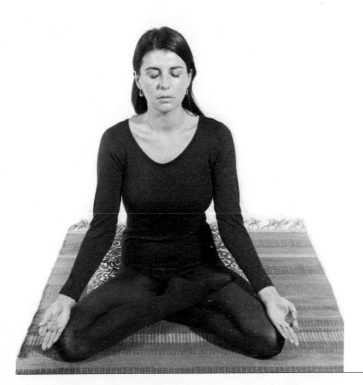

Do not permit the breath to gush or hiss in or out. Perform the inhalations and exhalations as quietly as possible. Think of the breathing as occurring more in the throat than the nostrils.

The counting is rhythmic and continuous; it is never interrupted. Once the counting begins, you keep it going like a metronome, steady and rhythmic.

Throughout the exercise, your attention must be fully focused on the counting. It must not become automatic while your attention is allowed to wander. Total concentration on the counting, in conjunction with respiration, is the seed for this meditation practice.

When the student has balanced the positive-negative currents and, as a result, is experiencing a state of deep quietude, he senses that his true nature, that which he really IS, lies beyond the positive-negative condition, beyond duality. All is ONE. Following completion of the 7 rounds, remain seated quietly for a short interval, and become aware of this ONENESS. (Fig. 149.)

Open your eyes and slowly extend your legs.

This terminates the meditation practice for today. (Make your notes.)

(Tomorrow's meditation practice requires a candle and holder. Have these on hand for tomorrow's session.)

19th day

Candle (2)

The value of Candle Meditation was outlined on the 2nd Day. At that time, we utilized the flame both as an introduction to visualization and as an expedient for impressing the element of *light* upon the consciousness.

On the 2nd Day, our visualization practice was concerned with simply retaining the image of the flame exactly as it was seen externally. But today, during visualization, we will *move* the flame; we will first decrease and then increase both its size and luminosity. Finally, we will attempt to merge with it.

Today's meditation requires a lighted candle. Place the candle (in its holder) and a match in your meditation area prior to beginning today's Hatha Yoga routine.

Instructions

Perform Hatha Yoga Intermediate Routine A page 91

Open your eyes.

Light the candle and place it approximately 2 feet from where you will be seated. Resume the cross-legged position.

Fix your gaze on the flame and hold it there steadily (blinking as necessary) for 5 minutes. Both your gaze and attention must remain fully fixed on the flame. (Fig. 150.)

When 5 minutes have elapsed, close your eyes and place your palms over them. (The candle remains lighted.)

Retain the image of the flame. When it becomes clear and steady, attempt to have it *recede* very slowly. Move it away from you into the distance until it becomes just a pinpoint of light. This must be done *very slowly* to help develop your control of the image and your ability in visualization. (Fig. 151.)

150. Full attention is focused on the flame for 5 minutes.

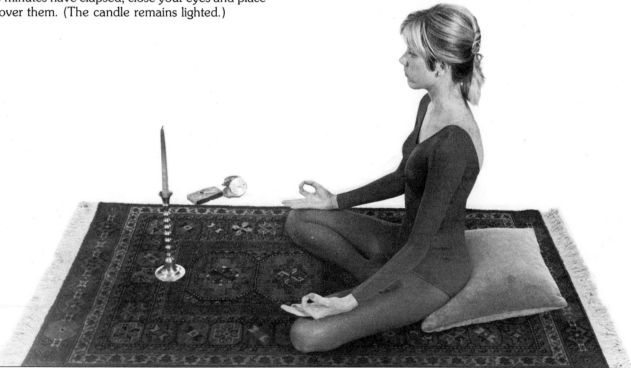

19th day

When you have moved the flame to this pinpoint distance, begin to bring it back toward you. Continue to move the flame very slowly into the foreground. As it is brought forward, it increases in size and luminosity. (Fig. 151.)

Continue to move it toward you until it is so large and so bright that the flame engulfs you. You merge with it and your consciousness is flooded with a light of great intensity. In this mergence, you terminate the subject-object relationship. There is no longer a "you" (subject) who is visualizing a "flame" (object). Your identity is no longer separate from that of the flame; you *become* the flame and *effect* Yoga with it. Now you and the flame are ONE, and in this ONENESS there is no "you" and no "flame." There simply IS.

Attempt to maintain this condition of ONENESS for the remaining minutes of the session. Initially, you will probably be able to remain in this state for only a brief period, but even a few seconds will be a highly meaningful experience. Whenever this Yogic state dissolves during your practice, the subject-object condition will return, and you once again exist as an "I" who is perceiving a "flame." When this occurs, attempt to merge again with the flame. This is best accomplished by opening your eyes and gazing briefly at the candle. Then palm your eyes and repeat the procedure of slowly moving the flame to the pinpoint distance and returning it to the place where the merger is effected.

When the 5 minutes that we allot to this visualization practice have elapsed, open your eyes and slowly extend your legs.

This terminates the meditation practice for today. (Make your notes.)

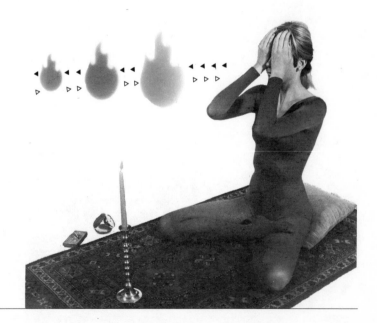

151. The flame is made to move. It decreases in size and luminosity when moved into the background, and increases in size and luminosity when brought to the foreground where a merger (Yoga) is effected.

20th day
OM (3)

The Yogi who utilizes OM as his primary seed for meditation gradually develops the ability to intone it silently and *continuously*. Even amidst daily activities he hears the OM sound. It becomes the constant undertone in his life. The mantra acts to dissolve the self so that his true nature, that of SELF, emerges.

We have learned the method for intoning OM audibly (6th and 13th Days). Now we must practice to also produce it internally, silently. In addition to being a highly effective technique for the meditation session, the internal intonation becomes applicable in active situations: riding on a bus, walking in the street, waiting in an office, and the like. Rather than the aimless, unfruitful thinking that usually occurs in these situations, turn the restless, agitated mind inward and hear the sound of OM. (This can be done with the eyes open or closed.) We will learn the silent OM technique today.

OM provides insulation against all types of emotional and mental disturbances and produces a profound serenity. Therefore, each moment you devote to this supreme mantra is time well invested.

Perform Hatha Yoga Intermediate Routine B page 99

Remain in the cross-legged posture. Your eyelids are partially lowered.

Exhale deeply.

In a count of 4 (approximating seconds), inhale deeply and quietly.

In a firm, steady, controlled voice, produce the sound "Oh" from the back of your mouth. (Fig. 152.) This should be performed in a count of 4.

Without interruption, continue the "Oh" sound, but now let it proceed from the front of your mouth. As it moves to the front, it assumes a slightly nasal quality. (Fig. 153.) This second sound is also performed in a count of 4.

Without interruption, press your lips together and produce the sound "Mmmm." (Fig. 154.) This sound should resonate strongly, like the buzzing of a bee, and you should feel the vibrations throughout your head and chest. Perform this in a count of 8.

Keep your lips together and *silently* complete the exhalation so that your lungs are emptied during an additional count of 2.

Without interruption, inhale deeply and quietly in a count of 4, and repeat the mantra. Devote 4 minutes to *japa* (repetition). You will be able to perform approximately 11 repetitions during this period.

When the 4 minutes have elapsed, continue the identical *japa,* but *silently,* for an additional 4 minutes. Everything remains identical: the counting, the inhalation, the intonation, the exhalation, but now the sound proceeds from the internal voice and is heard with the internal ear. Obviously, this internal technique requires your constant and total attention. (If you lose the sound, or if your attention wanders, simply perform the inhalation and begin again.) You will perform approximately 11 repetitions during this second 4-minute period. (See Summary page 144)

When the 4 minutes have elapsed, sit very quietly for an additional 2 minutes and become aware of what is transpiring within. Focus your attention fully on what you are experiencing as a result of your practice, and do not allow your mind to wander.

When the 2 minutes have elasped, open your eyes and slowly extend your legs.

This terminates the meditation practice for today. (Make your notes).

152. The "Oh" sound proceeds from back of mouth; lips in "o" shape.

153. "Oh" sound is transferred to front of mouth and has slight nasal quality; lips remain in "o" shape.

154. Lips together; strong vibrations of "Mmmm" throughout head and chest.

155. Silent intonation.

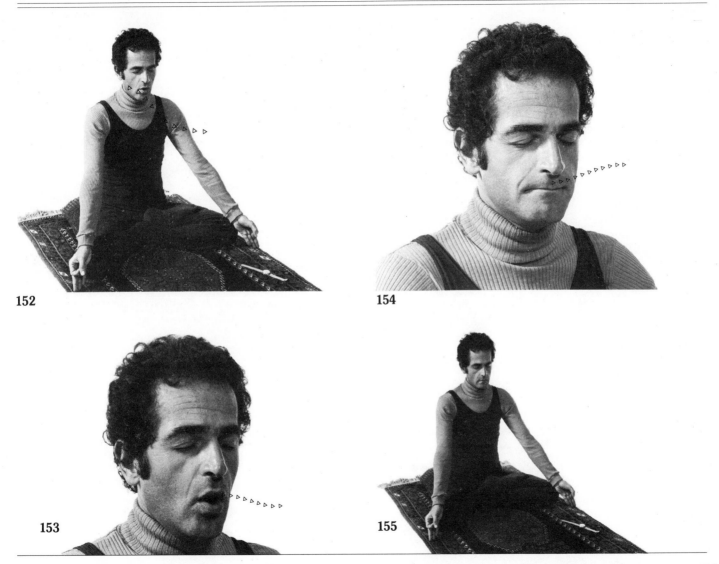

152

153

154

155

20th day

Summary

First 4-Minute Period

	Deep inhalation	"Oh"	"Oh"	"Mmmm"	Finish exhalation
Sound characteristics	Silent	Proceeds from back of mouth; lips in "o" shape	Transferred to front of mouth; has slight nasal quality; lips remain in "o" shape	Lips together; strong resonance vibrating throughout head and chest	Silent
Time (attempt to approximate seconds)	4	4	4	8	2

Second 4-Minute Period

Everything is identical with the above, but the *japa* is performed *silently* through the internal voice and the internal ear.

The rhythm remains steady: an uninterrupted 4, 4-4-8, 2.
Fix this rhythm firmly in your mind before beginning the practice.

The voice is steady, firm, controlled, and remains on the same pitch.

The attention is fully focused on both the external and internal sound.

21st day

Yantra (5)

The six-pointed star is the yantra contained within the heart center (*anahata chakra*). Fig. 156 depicts the location of the chakras in the etheric body; in an ascending order, the heart center is the fourth of the six chakras. For the beginning student, there is particular value in meditating upon those two yantras which represent the *heart* and *mind* centers. The heart center—today's seed for meditation—is the focal point of universal love and compassion, and these qualities manifest in and through the meditator as he continues to direct his consciousness there. The etheric heart center is situated to the right of the physical heart; it is in that area of the chest where a person points when he indicates "I" or "me."

The heart yantra is more complex than the previous yantras we have utilized for meditation. It is visualized first in its fundamental form, then it is encompassed by a circle and an additional inverted triangle is placed within its center.

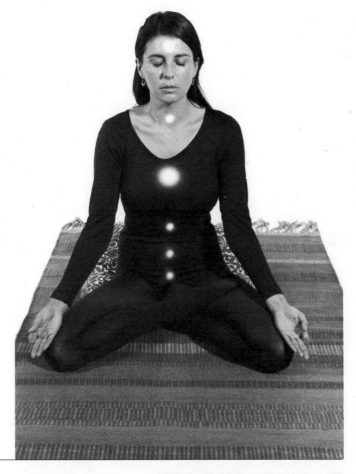

156. The location of the six *chakras* (center) in the etheric body. The heart center, fourth in the ascending order, is the seat of universal love.

Perform Hatha Yoga Intermediate Routine C page 107

Remain in the cross-legged posture. Open your eyes.

Place the book in a position where you may comfortably fix your gaze on Fig. 157.*

Previously, you directed your eyes along the various lines of the yantras to assist you in intensifying the impression. Today, however, attempt to gain the impression of the yantra in its entirety without dissecting it, without constructing it.

*If you had to come out of the cross-legged posture to properly position the book, resume the posture before beginning meditation practice.

Therefore, hold your gaze steadily and absorb the total yantra during a 2-minute period. Your attention must not wander.

Now close your eyes and visualize the identical figure for 3 minutes. No thoughts should enter your mind. If the image begins to fade, or if you perceive that your attention has wandered, remanifest the figure by an intensified visualization effort. If necessary, reinforce the image by opening your eyes and observing the figure on the page for a few additional moments. Then close your eyes and continue the visualization.

When the 3 minutes have elapsed, open your eyes.

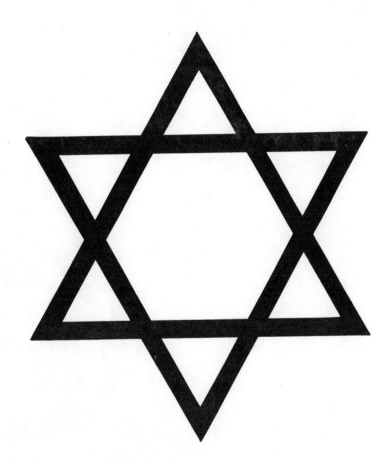

157. The yantra of the heart chakra.

21st day

Fix your gaze on Fig. 159. You will note that the figure is now encompassed by a circle and that there is the addition of an inverted triangle in its center. Hold your gaze steadily on this figure for 2 minutes.

When the 2 minutes have elapsed, close your eyes and visualize the identical figure for 3 minutes. The above instructions for visualization also apply here.

When the 3 minutes have elapsed, open your eyes and slowly extend your legs.

This terminates the meditation practice for today. (Make your notes.)

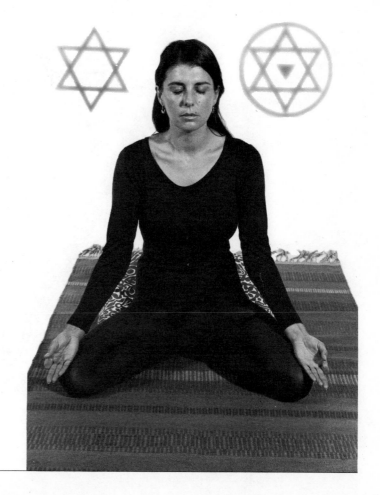

158. The fundamental (left) and more complex yantras are visualized successively.

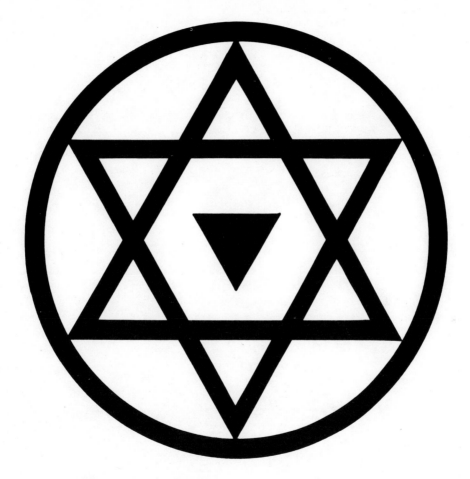

159. The fundamental yantra encompassed by a circle and containing an additional inverted triangle in its center.

Hatha Yoga

ADVANCED ROUTINE A

For Use on Days 22, 25, 28

According to your ability, you may either perform these advanced positions or remain with the elementary or intermediate positions and work toward the gradual accomplishment of this advanced practice. Your body will advise you of the best procedure in each *asana*. You must never strain or experience persistent discomfort in Hatha Yoga.

It may be that you are able to perform the advanced positions of some *asanas* but still only the elementary or intermediate positions of others. This is perfectly satisfactory. Simply continue to work toward the gradual accomplishment of the more advanced positions in each *asana*.

Remember that you begin each *asana* in the starting position learned in the Elementary Routines.

chest expansion

160. The upright position.

161. The extreme backward bend position. Arms are held as far from trunk as possible, knees remain straight, and eyes look upward. Do not retain breath. Hold motionless for 5.

162. The forward bend. Note that arms are now almost parallel to floor. Forehead is close to knees and may eventually touch them. Knees are straight and neck is limp. Hold motionless for 10.

Slowly straighten to upright position and repeat once.

Unclasp hands and gracefully lower yourself into seated position.

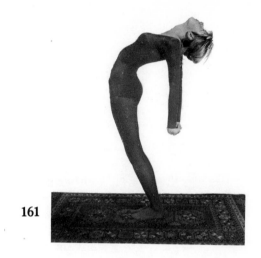

161

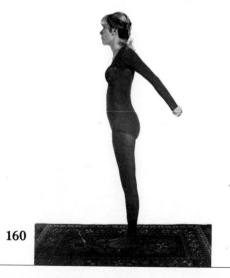

160

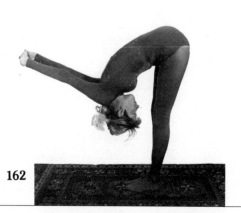

162

knee-and-thigh stretch

163. The beginning position.

164. You may now be able to lower knees an increased distance so that they are close to or touch floor. Hold trunk erect and maintain extreme stretch for a count of 10.

Relax hands and arms for a few moments. During this relaxation, knees can be raised. Repeat. Perform 3 times.

Unclasp hands. Move gracefully into a lying position. Stomach and forehead rest on mat.

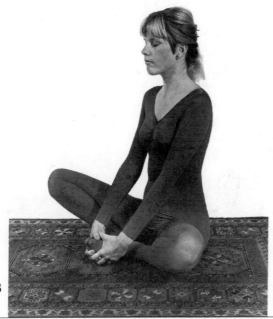

163

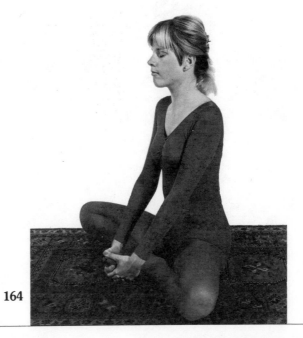

164

cobra

165. Keep arms at sides and very slowly raise trunk as high as possible.

166. When you have reached your limit, gracefully bring hands up and place them in the usual position beneath shoulders.
In very slow motion, continue to raise trunk with hands now pushing against floor. Head bends far backward and spine is continually curved. Fig. 166

depicts the completed posture. Elbows are now straight. Hold without motion for 10.

Very slowly lower trunk halfway to floor. When this halfway position is reached, smoothly and gracefully bring arms back to sides so that back muscles must support trunk.
Continue to *slowly* lower trunk until forehead rests on mat. Relax a few moments and repeat. Perform 3 times. Relax with forehead on mat.

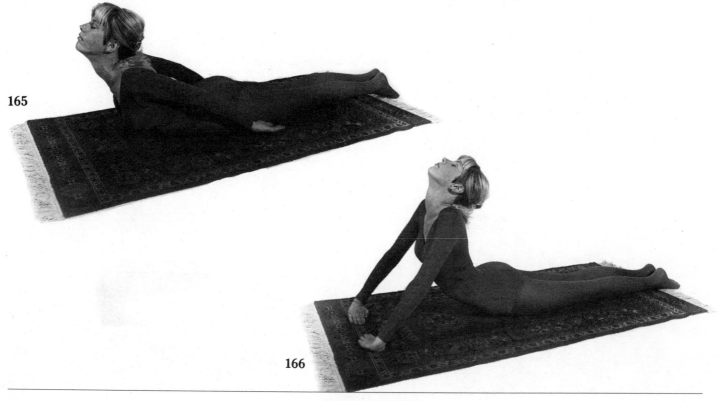

165

166

head twist

167– There are no advanced positions for the Head Twist.
168. Perform the movements as previously, holding the extreme position of each for a count of 20.

Do the routine twice.

Rest chin on mat and lower arms to sides.

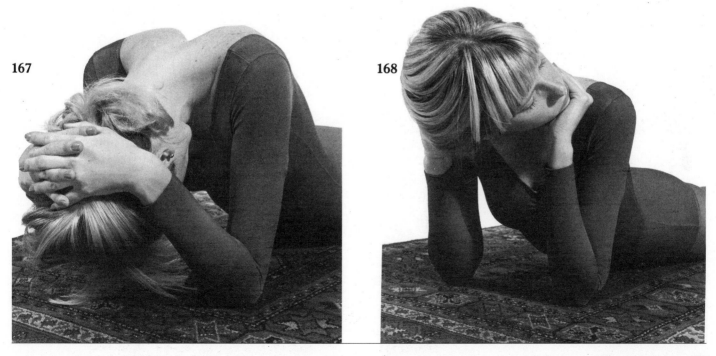

167

168

bow

169. The beginning position.

170. The extreme position. Eyes look upward and knees are as close together as possible. Breathe normally. Hold without motion for 10. Lower knees and chin to floor slowly, but retain the hold on feet.

Pause a few moments and repeat. Perform 3 times. Following final repetition, release feet and lower them slowly to floor. Rest cheek on mat and relax.

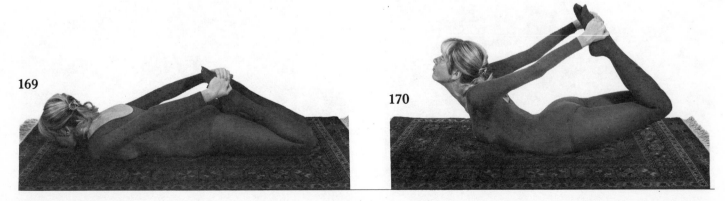

169

170

Observation of the Breath

Sit in cross-legged posture and observe the breath for 1 minute as instructed on page 21.

Hatha Yoga

ADVANCED ROUTINE B

For Use on Days 23, 26, 29

All starting positions are identical with those learned in Elementary Routine B.

rishi's posture

171. Trunk and arms turned left to the 90-degree position.

172. Right hand takes a firm hold on back of ankle or heel while gaze follows left hand to upright position illustrated. Hold without motion for 10.

Slowly raise trunk, bring extended arms into frontward position. Twist slowly to right and perform the identical movements. Perform 3 times to each side, alternating left-right.

Following final repetition, slowly lower arms to sides and relax.

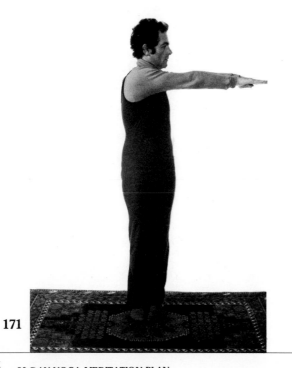

171

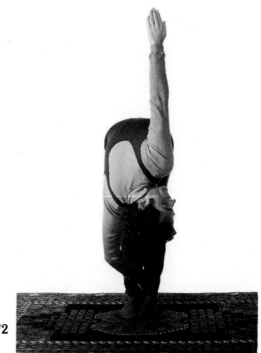

172

balance posture

173. Perform the intermediate position. Hold for 5.

174. Very slowly and gracefully bring right foot up and back; simultaneously lower left arm so that it is parallel to floor. Hold with as little motion as possible for 5.

Slowly lower foot to floor and arms to sides.

Perform the identical movements on opposite side.

Perform 3 times on each side, alternating sides.

Following final repetition, lower yourself gracefully into a seated position on mat.

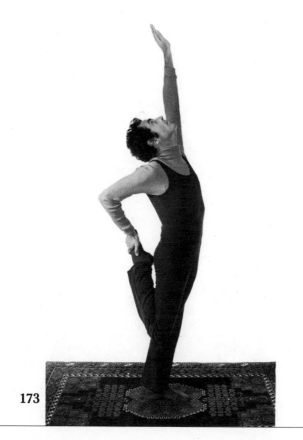

173

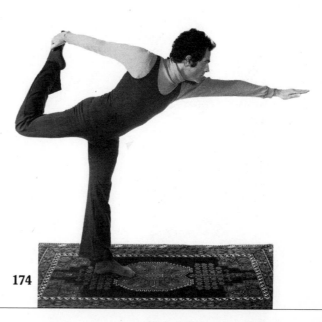

174

alternate leg stretch

175. In the beginning position, trunk bends backward as far as possible. Head is back and eyes look upward.

176. During slow-motion dive, trunk comes forward a sufficient distance so that both hands may hold left foot. Trunk is lowered as far as possible and forehead comes close to or actually rests on knee. Elbows are lowered toward floor. Relax body as much as possible. Hold without motion for 10.

Slowly straighten trunk to upright position.

Raise arms slowly and repeat the movements. Perform 3 times.

Perform the identical movements 3 times with right leg extended.

Following final repetition, extend left leg and rest hands on thighs.

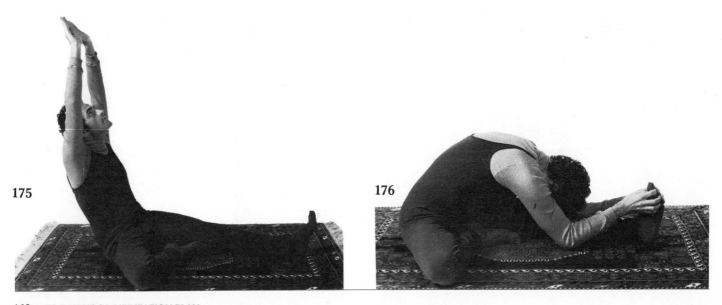

175

176

backward bend

177. Begin as usual with top of feet on floor, but then change the position so that toes rest on floor. Knees remain together throughout the movements.

178. Cautiously inch backward on fingertips as far as possible. Place palms firmly on floor. Arms are parallel with sides. Slowly arch trunk upward as far as possible and lower head backward as far as possible. Remain seated on heels.

Work toward a hold of 20 seconds. (This *asana* is performed only once.) Slowly raise head, inch forward on fingertips, and return to starting position of Fig. 177.

Come off heels, swing legs around, and extend them straight outward.

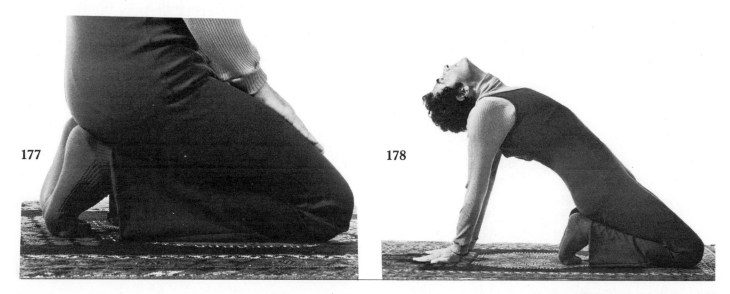

177

178

twist

179. The position prior to the Twist.

180–
181. As you begin twisting trunk to left, remove left hand from floor and hold right side of waist. Turn trunk and head as far to left as possible. Hold without motion for 10.

Place left hand back down on floor and slowly turn trunk frontward. Maintain the hold on knee. Relax a few moments. Repeat twisting of trunk. Perform 3 twists.

Following final repetition, turn frontward, extend both legs.

Perform the identical movements on right side by exchanging the words "left" and "right" in the above directions. Perform 3 times to right side.

Following final repetition, turn frontward, extend both legs, and assume cross-legged posture.

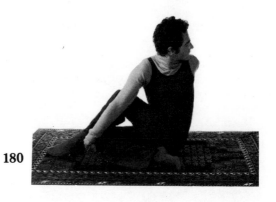

180

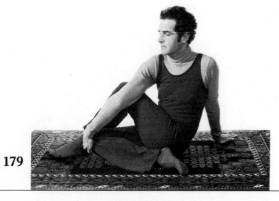

179

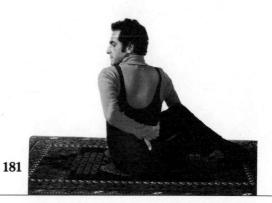

181

Observation of the Breath

Sit in cross-legged posture and observe the breath for 1 minute as instructed on page 21.

Hatha Yoga

ADVANCED ROUTINE C

For Use on Days 24, 27, 30

All starting positions are identical with
those learned in Elementary Routine C.

triangle

182. Move legs gracefully into a wide stance and raise arms to shoulder level.

183. Slowly bend to left and hold left ankle. Pull on ankle and lower trunk so that it is parallel with floor. Bring right arm over head (with elbow straight) so that it is also in the parallel position. Knees must remain straight. Hold for 10.

Slowly straighten to upright position of Fig. 182.

Execute the identical movements to right.

Perform 3 times to each side, alternating left-right.

Following final repetition, bring arms to sides, gracefully draw legs together, and lower yourself into a seated position on mat.

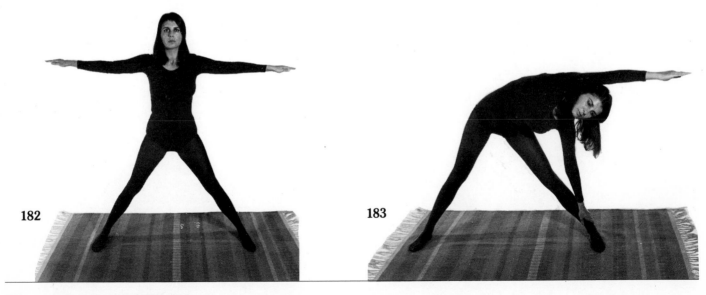

182

183

back stretch

184. Extend both legs straight outward. In very slow motion, raise arms to overhead position and bend backward as far as possible. Look upward.

185. During slow-motion forward dive, trunk comes forward a sufficient distance so that hands may hold feet.

Pull against feet and slowly lower trunk as far as possible without strain. In the extreme position, forehead rests on knees, and elbows and forearms are close to or touch floor. Although the stretch is extreme, body remains relaxed. Hold without motion for 10.

Slowly straighten trunk to upright position.

Raise arms slowly and repeat the movements. Perform 3 times.

Following final repetition, straighten trunk to upright position, rest hands on thighs, and slowly lower back to floor.

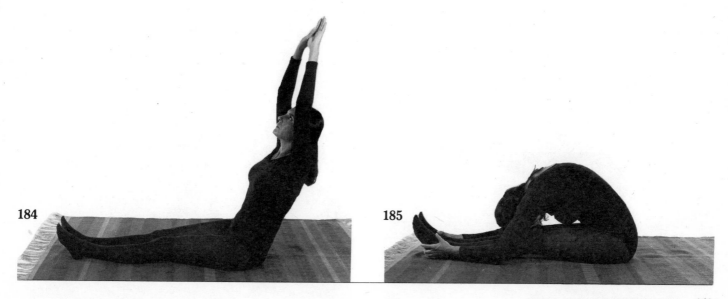

184

185

shoulder stand

186. Bring legs back gracefully over head.

187. Straighten trunk and legs to the completed position. Trunk is now totally vertical and at a direct right angle with head. Chin is pressed against top of chest. Body is straight but relaxed. Breathe normally. Hold for 1–3 minutes.

Slowly lower legs behind head for the Plough *asana*.

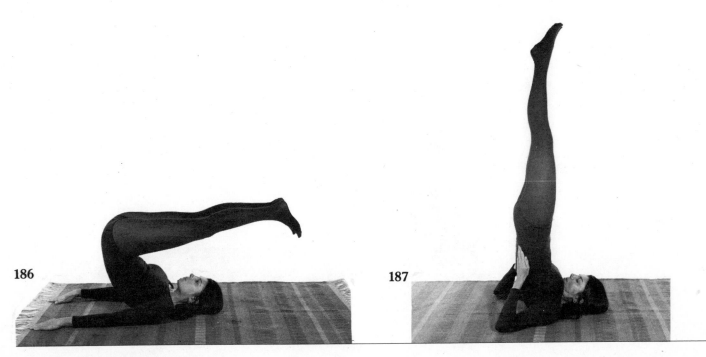

186

187

plough

188. The completed intermediate position.
Hold for 30 seconds.

189. Bring arms up from sides and clasp them on top of
head. You will now be able to inch back with toes a
short but very significant distance. (The emphasis is
transferred from lower to middle area of back.) Knees
remain straight. Hold without motion for 30 seconds.

Bring arms back to sides and place palms against
floor. The procedure for coming out of the position is
the same as in the previous routines. Relax a few
moments in prone position and then come into seated
cross-legged posture.

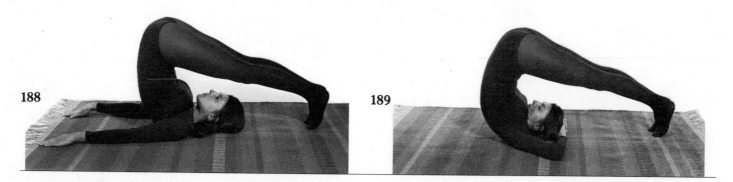

188

189

head roll

190– There are no advanced positions for the Head Roll.

191. Perform the movements as previously,
holding each of the four positions for a
count of 10. Do the routine twice.

Upon completion, remain in cross-legged posture,
keep eyes closed and raise head.

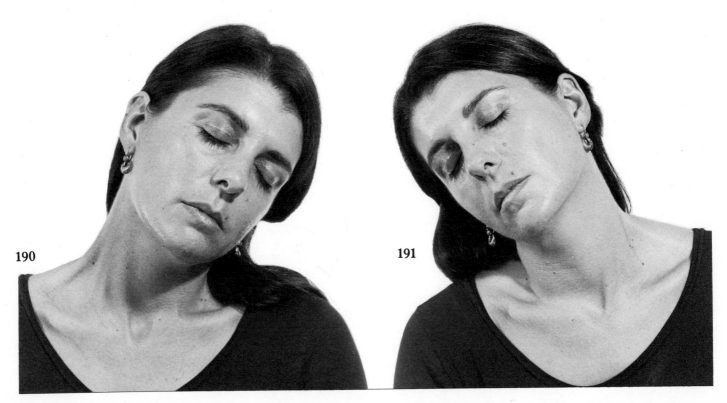

190

191

Observation of the Breath

Sit in cross-legged posture and observe the breath for 1 minute as instructed on page 21.

22nd day

Visualization of Perfect Health During Deep Relaxation

The ordinary person believes that he exists in a world that is *real,* one that is external to or apart from him, in which he finds himself without knowing why or from where he has come. His life is usually spent in a continual subject-object relationship with this world: he perceives his situation as one in which there is an "I," an "ego" that he refers to as "me" (subject), and that this "me" exists in a world (object) where it must undertake whatever is necessary for its survival. The fact that this is not the case, that the world is not an entity separate from the "I," but that the "I" projects the universe and that all things he believes he is sensing in a real, external world are, in reality, *flowing through him,* comes as a revelation of the first magnitude. Through regular, serious meditation, the student gradually perceives that he is existing in a world, or dimension, formed entirely by his thoughts. He realizes that he is manifesting or projecting his world as the movie projector transmits the film onto the screen, and then proceeds to search for his happiness and fulfillment in this projection as though it were real! This realization leads the student to additional profound realizations. He understands, for example, that just as a person may project his universe, so may he withdraw it. Indeed, a number of the techniques we are utilizing are concerned exactly with such withdrawal.

The beginning student usually conceives of withdrawal in terms of pulling back from a real, objective world. But the more advanced meditator recognizes that he does not retreat from the world, like a snail retires into its shell, but that *he totally withdraws his universe and that no real, objective world remains apart from him once this withdrawal occurs.* This fact is perceived in the course of continued practice.

The physical organism, the body, is an aspect of the world that man projects. And just as his thoughts and visualizations, consciously applied in a particular manner, will influence his world accordingly, so do they have their effect on his body. Although the Yoga student grows to understand that attempting to consciously alter the world he projects is *not* to his advantage (actually, any such attempt will retard his progress in the attainment of Self-realization and is therefore strongly discouraged by the guru), there is no objection, in the beginning stages of this practice, to promoting the health and well-being of the *body* through visualization. The pertinent technique is the seed of today's practice.

Innumerable students have extolled the effectiveness of this technique as it relates to the maintenance and restoration of health. But its greater value lies in the fact that the student, in experiencing that *he becomes what he thinks and visualizes,* begins to understand that he, himself, is entirely responsible for any and all situations in which he finds himself. He recognizes the illusory nature of destiny, luck, and fortune, and this recognition leads him more and more to turn inward, to examine the nature of his thoughts and to trace them to their source. It is at this source—the place from which the thoughts arise, and not in the world they project—that his fulfillment lies.

Instructions

Perform Hatha Yoga Advanced Routine A page 151

From the cross-legged posture, slowly extend your legs straight outward.

Slowly lower your back to the floor.

Place your arms as illustrated in Fig. 192. Palms face upward. Close your eyes. Breathe normally.

Allow your body to become limp.

The procedure is identical with that of the 1st and 15th Days. Beginning with your feet, direct your consciousness very slowly and very deliberately through your body, relaxing each area in turn: feet, calves, thighs, buttocks, groin, abdomen, chest, back; then down to your hands and up through your arms, shoulders, neck, jaw, and face. (If you have any doubts regarding this procedure, do not hesitate to refer to the instructions of the 1st and 15th Days.)

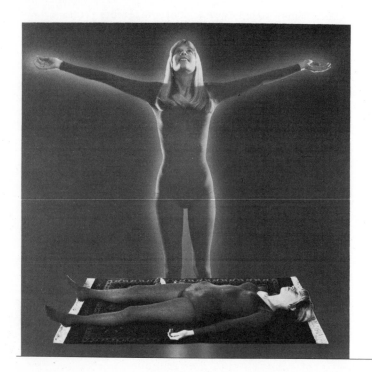

192. An image of joy and radiance is manifested while the body remains in the totally relaxed state.

22nd day

Remain in the relaxed condition for several moments and observe your breathing.

Now, to be certain that you have allowed each set of muscles to let go completely so that the ultimate state of relaxation is attained, repeat the exercise. Therefore, once again, very slowly and deliberately direct your consciousness through your entire body, becoming acutely sensitive to all areas that may have remained tensed, however slightly.

When your attention has moved into your facial area for the second time, approximately 5 minutes will have elapsed, and your body should be in the totally relaxed state.

Now *visualize your body in a state of perfect health.* Fig. 192 depicts one possible image for this objective. The meditator is visualizing herself in a joyous, radiant state that, to her, represents perfect health. You may visualize yourself in this same attitude or in any position and environment that, for you, is representative of a condition of well-being.

Remaining in the totally relaxed state with your eyes closed, form your image. Once formed, surround it with an aura of white light, brilliant and vibrating. Maintain your visualization steadily for approximately 5 minutes. The aura of white light that is emanating from the figure remains brilliant and vibrating. If the image fades, or disappears, it must be remanifested.

(If you are afflicted with an illness, visualize your body in a stationary position with the afflicted area[s] radiating light for the entire 5-minute period. If you have a condition that affects your back, visualize your figure, standing and stationary, from a back view, and see the light radiating from the afflicted area of your back for the 5-minute period. If you are ill, or recovering from an illness, this technique may be employed several times each day without the Hatha Yoga routine indicated for today's practice.)

When the 5 minutes have elapsed, open your eyes, slowly raise your trunk and come into a seated position.

This terminates the meditation practice for today. (Make your notes.)

23rd day
Active Meditation (2)

On the 13th Day, we explained how the intonation of OM is symbolic of the creation, preservation, dissolution, and withdrawal of the universe. Today, by including an additional element in Active Meditation, and altering the imagery from that of the 9th Day, this identical cycle—creation, preservation, dissolution, withdrawal—is simulated. Therefore, in performing the movements of today's Active Meditation, you place yourself in concord with the eternal cosmological cycle and, consequently, with the ONE through which the cycle moves. This concordance is Yoga.

Perform Hatha Yoga Advanced Routine B page 159

Come into a standing position.

193. Exhale deeply and allow your trunk to relax as depicted. This stance represents an attitude of depletion. A minimum of life-force is present. The universe is unborn in its potential state. Feel and visualize this passive condition. (Your eyes may be open or partially closed—whichever you find more conducive to manifesting the indicated conditions.)

194. Begin a very deep, very slow inhalation. As you inhale, expand your abdomen to permit the air to enter your lower lungs.

Begin to raise your arms slowly, palms up, elbows straight. As life-force (*prana*) enters your lungs, the organism is activated and stirs. The creation is in its initial stage. Feel and visualize this birth of activity.

195. Continue the deep, slow inhalation and the slow raising of your arms with your elbows straight. (If the inhalation is not performed very slowly and very deeply, it will be completed before you can perform the necessary physical movements or have the opportunity for adequate visualization.) Now your chest expands, and as more air enters your lungs and more life-force fills your body, you become increasingly alive. The creation continues.

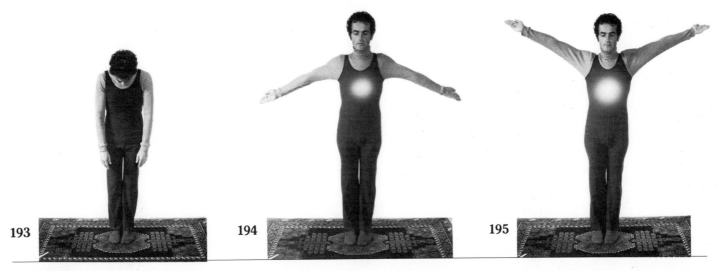

193   194   195

196. As your palms meet overhead, the inhalation, representing the creation, is completed. Now your lungs are full, your chest is expanded, your abdomen is slightly contracted. Retain the air for a count of 5. During this breath retention, feel and visualize your body permeated with *prana* and totally vitalized. This is the preservation stage of the cycle.

197. Begin a very slow exhalation. The movements are now reversed. Your arms are slowly lowered, palms turned down, elbows straight. As the exhalation continues, the life-force is gradually depleted, and your trunk becomes increasingly limp. The stage of dissolution is now manifesting. Feel and visualize this pro-gressive depletion. (If the exhalation is not controlled, it will be completed before you have had the opportunity for adequate visualization or time to perform the necessary movements.)

When the exhalation is completed, your arms rest once again at your sides, and the organism should be felt and visualized in the totally depleted, passive state. The dissolution is complete. Suspend your breath so that no air enters your empty lungs for several seconds. The universe is now withdrawn, at rest, potential. (Fig. 193.)

Repeat the *asana*. Devote 7 minutes to Active Meditation. During this period, you will be able to perform approximately 10 repetitions.

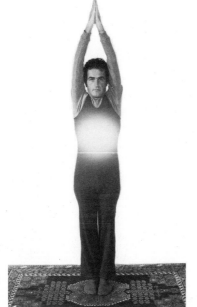

196

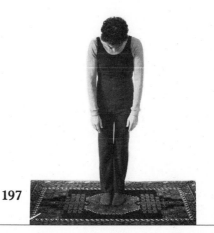

197

23rd day

At the end of the 7-minute period, lower yourself gracefully to the floor and assume the cross-legged posture. Close your eyes.

During the following 3 minutes, become aware of what is transpiring within. Focus your attention fully on what you are experiencing, and do not allow your mind to wander.

When the 3 minutes have elapsed, open your eyes and slowly extend your legs.

This terminates the meditation practice for today. (Make your notes.)

24th day
White Light (Healing)

On the 3rd Day, we employed the White Light for revitalization. Today, it will be utilized as an element for healing.

In what we may refer to as the "physiology of Hatha Yoga," health and well-being are defined in terms of an adequate supply and the normal circulation of *prana*. It is partially to help ensure these that Hatha Yoga is practiced. If the pranic supply is reduced or its circulation impeded, various negative conditions develop, and health is impaired accordingly. All healing, regardless of the method or by whom it is applied, is a conscious or unconscious effort to normalize the pranic flow.

In today's meditation practice, we learn how to consciously direct *prana* to any area where a negative condition exists. The premise is that by increasing the supply of life-force at the point where it is needed, healing is promoted.

As you continue to gain aptitude—steadiness and strength—in visualization, the effectiveness of the White Light technique for both revitalization and healing will increase.

Perform Hatha Yoga Advanced Routine C page 167

Remain in the cross-legged posture. Close your eyes.

Let's assume you are experiencing tension, stiffness, and pain in your left shoulder. It is into this area, therefore, that you wish to direct additional *prana*.

Place all ten fingertips lightly on your solar plexus (the sun center; the third *chakra*). Exhale deeply.

Very slowly inhale deeply and fully. During this inhalation, visualize the pranic current as an intense white light. (Fig. 198.) It enters through your nostrils, moves downward into the region of your solar plexus, and passes into your fingertips where it remains. This is the continuous visualization during the entire *slow* inhalation. (Fig. 199.)

When the inhalation is completed, *retain the air* and transfer your ten fingertips to that area of your shoulder where you are experiencing the discomfort.

Very slowly exhale deeply and fully. During this exhalation, visualize the *prana*, the white light, flowing from your fingertips into your shoulder, flooding it with life-force. This is the continuous visualization during the entire *slow* exhalation. (Fig. 200.)

198

198. The white light (*prana*).

199. The course of the *prana* during the slow inhalation.

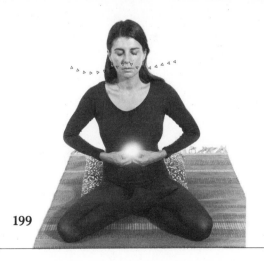

199

When the exhalation is completed, *suspend breathing* for a few moments while you slowly return your fingertips to your solar plexus.

Begin the inhalation and repeat the procedure.

Obviously, your attention must remain totally focused on the visualization of the white light throughout the practice. During the 10-minute period, you will be able to perform approximately 20 repetitions. However, if you wish to perform additional repetitions to increase the possibility of remedying the shoulder (or any other) condition, you should certainly do so. You can rest briefly, following the first 10 minutes of practice, and then repeat one or two more 10-minute periods. Additionally, you can repeat the practice at other times during the day.

Although we have used the shoulder as an example, *prana* may be directed to any part of the body. If an area of your back required *prana,* you could separate your hands and bring them around to the pertinent area from your left and right sides during retention of the air. Then during the exhalation, the white light is directed into the desired area, following which your fingertips are returned to your solar plexus during suspension of your breathing, and the process repeated. If, during an illness, you are unable to assume the cross-legged posture, the technique can be practiced in a reclining position. With a little consideration, you will be able to make whatever adjustments are necessary in any situation to accommodate the technique.

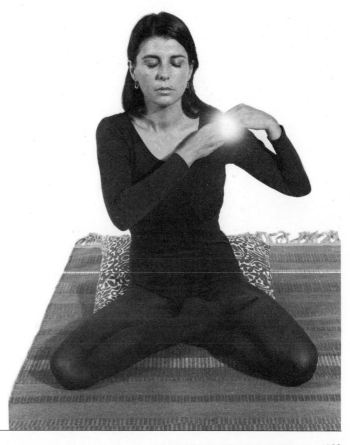

200. *Prana* is directed into the afflicted area during the slow exhalation.

24th day

When the 10-minute period has elapsed, keep your eyes closed, rest your hands (in the *mudra*) on your knees, and relax a few moments. Direct your consciousness to the afflicted area and become aware of any change that may have occurred there. (Fig. 201.)

Open your eyes and slowly extend your legs.

This terminates the meditation practice for today. (Make your notes.)

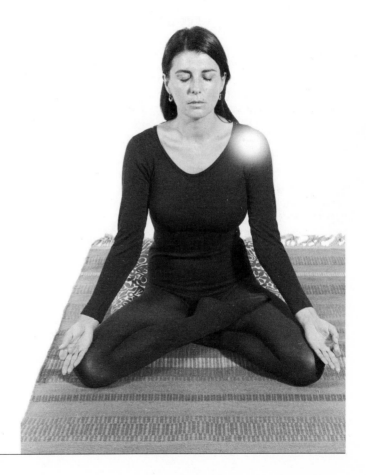

201. The increased supply of life-force remains in the afflicted area.

25th day
Yantra (6)

Today's yantra, the symbol of OM, is contained within the sixth center (*ajna chakra*). Fig. 202 depicts its location. This center is the seat of spiritual knowledge where the instruction of the guru is received. To gain access to such knowledge and instruction, the meditator directs his consciousness to this "third eye" center by visualizing the OM symbol. With his consciousness fixed there, the student learns how to listen for guidance. His listening is done with an inner ear that gradually becomes attuned and sensitive to the inner voice. At times, the instruction is readily available; at times, it is slow in coming. But the student understands this pattern and, when necessary, waits patiently because he knows it *will* be forthcoming.

The form that the inner instruction takes cannot be described; it is subtle, sublime, and totally transcends that knowledge which is usually sought by the ordinary mind. This is Knowledge and Understanding not of the transient, but of the Eternal.

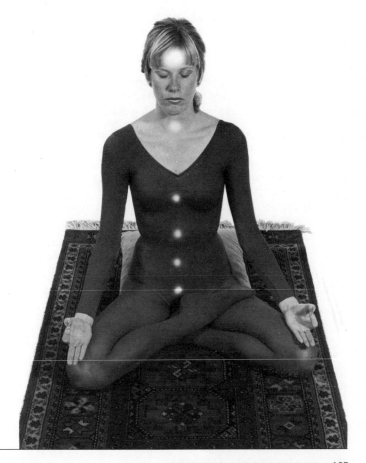

202. The location of the OM chakra, seat of spiritual knowledge, where the instruction of the guru is received.

Perform Hatha Yoga Advanced Routine A page 151

Remain in the cross-legged posture. Open your eyes.

Place the book in a position where you may comfortably fix your gaze on Fig. 204.*

Hold your gaze steadily on the figure for 5 minutes. (Today's practice is divided into two 5-minute segments.) Both your gaze and attention must remain fully fixed on the figure.

As was the case with the heart center (21st Day), we are no longer concerned with the individual configurations of the yantra, but absorb it in its entirety during the 5-minute period.

Now close your eyes and visualize the identical figure for 5 minutes. Do not allow your attention to wander; no thoughts should enter your mind. If the image begins to fade, or if you perceive that your attention has wandered, re-manifest the figure. If necessary, reinforce the image by opening your eyes and observing the figure on the page for a few additional moments. Then close your eyes and continue the visualization.

When the 5 minutes have elapsed, open your eyes and slowly extend your legs.

This terminates the meditation practice for today. (Make your notes.)

(Tomorrow's meditation practice requires an object for touching and feeling. Any small object that you may have found pleasing to your touch will be satisfactory. Have this on hand for tomorrow's session.)

*If you had to come out of the cross-legged posture to properly position the book, resume the posture before beginning meditation practice.

203. Visualization of OM.

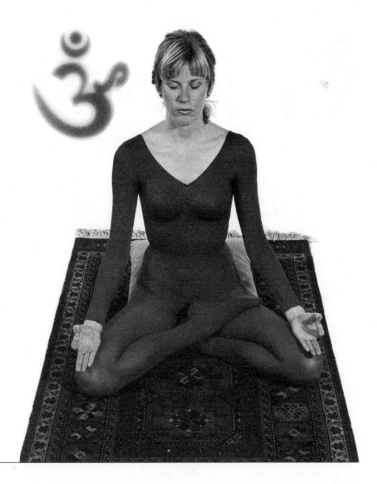

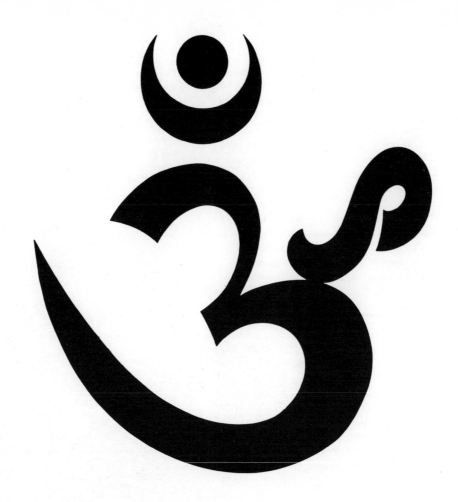

204. The symbol of OM.

26th day

Touch

Touch is another of the senses that has proven to be an excellent seed for meditation.

During the course of the day, we may touch hundreds of objects but actually *feel* very few. That is, we have only the most superficial encounter with the objects we touch; we seldom make the effort to really *contact* them, to become involved with them, to experience them as total entities.

Infants and youngsters derive much pleasure and knowledge from their tactile experiences, but adults, especially in the "civilized" countries, seem to become greatly desensitized in this area. The sense of touch has proven to be a fruitful seed for meditation, because as the student contacts and examines an object according to the instructions presented in today's practice, he once again becomes aware of what it is like to really *feel*. His fascination with this renewed awareness is conducive to becoming totally involved with aspects of touch during the practice session, and he is able to focus his attention in that intense, one-pointed manner which is a prerequisite to productive meditation. In this one-pointed state, he may find he can also effect that merger which has been a major objective in many of our previous sessions. In merging (Yoga), the student understands that by truly contacting one thing, he has contacted *all* things. But whether or not this merger occurs, the application of today's contact-feeling technique which, among other benefits, reawakens tactile awareness, will be of significant value: the experience that transpires during the practice period is extended to the activities of everyday life, and the student soon becomes sensitive to an entire dimension of his existence that formerly was largely obscured.

Today's meditation requires an object for touching and feeling. Any small object that you have previously found pleasing to your touch will be satisfactory. Place this object in your meditation area before beginning today's Hatha Yoga routine.

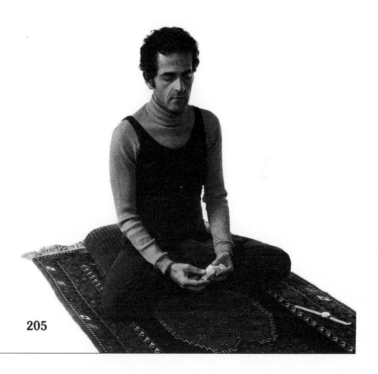

205

Perform Hatha Yoga Advanced Routine B page 159

Remain in the cross-legged posture. Open your eyes.

Pick up the object you have chosen and place it so that the fingers of both hands may feel it. (Figs. 205–206.)

Close your eyes.

During the next 10 minutes, fix your attention on this object and do not permit anything to distract it. Become totally involved with the object. Examine its qualities. Feel its weight, texture, shape, temperature. Take your time with each quality, and use both hands and as many fingers as possible in your investigation. Your concentration must be total. If you perceive that your attention has wandered, return it to the object and resume your examination.

You will be able to *merge* with the object to the extent that your concentration remains fixed. That is, if your mind and sense of touch have been totally involved with the object for several minutes without interruption, you begin to *become* that object. The subject-object relationship is terminated. There is no longer a "you" who is feeling an object; your identity is no longer separate from that of the object. You *become* the object and effect Yoga with it. You and the object are ONE, and in this ONENESS there is no "you" and there is no "object." There only IS.

Attempt to maintain this condition of ONENESS for the remainder of the session. Whenever this state dissolves during your practice, and the subject-object condition remanifests, attempt to merge again through the technique of total, unwavering concentration on the object.

When the 10 minutes have elapsed, open your eyes and slowly extend your legs.

This terminates the meditation practice for today. (Make your notes.)

205–
206. With the attention focused in the total, unwavering, one-pointed manner, the meditator merges, effects Yoga, with the object being contacted.

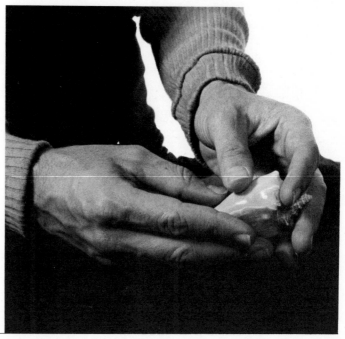

206

27th day

Asana Meditation (3)

You are now sufficiently familiar with the *asanas* of Routine C to utilize them as seeds for meditation. The technique is identical with that which we applied to Routine A on the 7th Day and Routine B on the 14th Day. The *asana* is converted from a physical exercise to a meditation practice by totally immersing the mind in the *feeling* of the movements, and by becoming aware of their effects on the areas of the body that are involved. Additionally, during the hold segment of the *asana,* the attention is directed to that area of the body where the maximum emphasis is experienced.

This technique focuses the mind in the one-pointed manner and, through intense concentration, also accelerates progress in the *asanas.* Upon completion of the course, you will be advised to utilize this technique in each of your Hatha Yoga routines so that the entire session, from the first to the last movement, becomes a form of meditation.

Perform Hatha Yoga Advanced Routine C page 167

Repeat the identical routine of Hatha Yoga *asanas* that you performed today. The postures will now be performed *with your total attention focused on all of the movements.* You are to *feel* their effects on the areas of the body that are involved.

The arrows indicate those particular areas of the body which receive the greatest emphasis during the hold. Direct your consciousness to the indicated area and maintain it there for the duration of the hold. If you detect that your attention is wandering, return it immediately to the movements or the hold.

Rest briefly between *asanas*. The number of repetitions for the *asanas* in this meditation routine differs from that of the regular routine.

Now stand up gracefully, turn your attention inward, and perform the routine.

207. Hold for 10 on each side. Perform twice to each side, alternating left-right.

208. Hold for 20. Perform twice.

209. Hold for 1 minute.

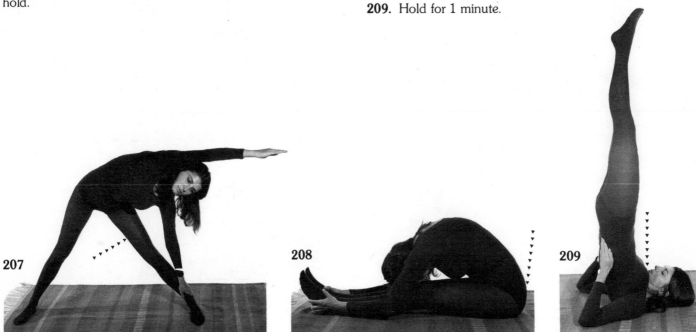

207   208   209

27th day

210. Hold the intermediate position for 1 minute.

211. Hold the advanced position for 1 minute.

212–
213. Hold each of the four positions for 20.

Upon completion of the routine, assume the cross-legged posture and rest for approximately 1 minute

with your eyes partially closed. Become aware of how your body feels at this point.

Open your eyes and slowly extend your legs.

This terminates the meditation practice for today. (Make your notes.)

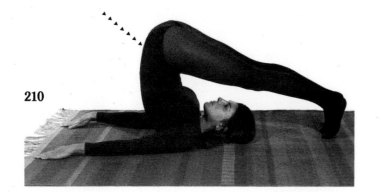

210

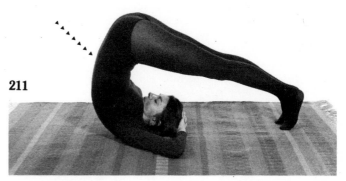

211

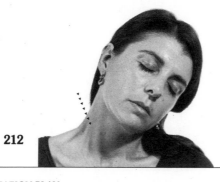

212

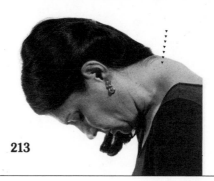

213

Hansa-Soham: The Involuntary Mantras

On three previous days, we intoned the mantra OM. Whether OM or any other mantra is intoned audibly or silently, it requires the student's full attention. Although the serious student practices for the mantra to infuse his being in such a way that it is sounded continually and becomes a constant undertone in all of his activities, in the initial stages mantra must be a totally *conscious* practice.

There are, however, two unconscious, automatic, and involuntary mantras that are inherent in the process of respiration: *each inhalation and each exhalation is a mantra!* The syllables of these mantras are *aham-sah,* "I am THAT" (THAT = SELF), and the converse, *sah-aham,* "THAT I am." The former is inherent in the inhalation and the latter in the exhalation. When applied to the inhalation, *aham-sah* assumes the sound of *hansa;* when applied to the exhalation, *sah-aham* assumes the sound of *soham.* (Each "a" is pronounced as in "Ah!")

Until today, Observation of the Breath preceded meditation practice. Today, Observation of the Breath *is the seed for* meditation. Rather than simply observing the breath—focusing the attention on the process and rhythm of breathing—we now direct the inner ear to hear the sounds inherent in respiration. We *hear* the mantras *hansa, soham,* "I am THAT," "THAT I am." This practice makes the student consciously aware that he is performing unconscious *japa* as he breathes, and that he is automatically reaffirming—approximately 15 times each minute, or 21,600 times each day—the fact that he is always in the state of Yoga, that there can be no separation from the ONE.

In order of importance, *hansa-soham* is considered second only to OM. OM is the supreme one-syllable mantra. *Hansa-soham* are the supreme two-syllable mantras.

**Perform Hatha Yoga Advanced Routine A page 151. Observation of the Breath
is the seed for today's meditation practice and is therefore eliminated from
the Hatha Yoga routine. Proceed from the Bow *asana* directly to meditation.**

Assume the cross-legged posture. Lower your eyelids.
Breathe normally.

Direct your attention to your breathing and simply
observe the inhalations and exhalations as you have done
previously. Continue this observation for 3 minutes.

Now direct your inner ear to *hear* the respiration mantras. Hear *hansa,* ("I am That") during the inhalation and
soham, ("That I am") during the exhalation. Each "a" is
heard as in "Ah!"

These mantras are *heard* with the inner ear. Your lips do
not move. Obviously, your attention must remain totally fixed
on the syllables. Continue this conscious *japa* for the remaining 7 minutes of the session.

When the 7 minutes have elapsed, open your eyes and
slowly extend your legs.

This terminates the meditation practice for today. (Make
your notes.)

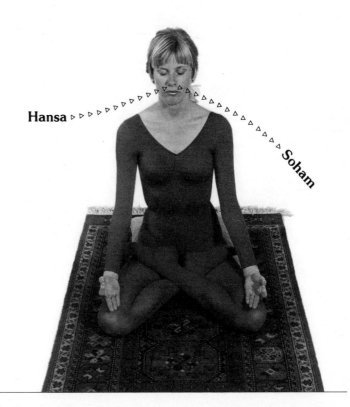

214. The involuntary mantras. *Hansa* is inherent
in inhalation and *soham* in exhalation.

29th day
Alternate Nostril Breathing (4)

Today, we will practice Alternate Nostril Breathing in its completed form.

To inhalation, retention, and exhalation we now add a fourth segment: suspension. It occurs at the end of each exhalation when the lungs are empty and is maintained for a count of 4. Therefore, the final rhythm is 4-16-8-4; this is a demanding rhythm but will prove to be the most effective in slowing the breathing, quieting the mind, and conditioning the consciousness to transcend the ego.

Perform Hatha Yoga Advanced Routine B page 159

215 –
216. Remain in the cross-legged posture with your left hand in the *mudra*. Keep your eyes partially closed (only a slit of light should enter at the bottom).

Place the tip of your right thumb lightly against your right nostril and your ring and little fingers lightly against your left. Your index and middle fingers are together, and they rest lightly on your forehead (the "third eye" area).

Slowly and as quietly as possible exhale deeply through both nostrils.

217. When the exhalation is completed, immediately close your right nostril by pressing your thumb against it. Slowly and quietly inhale deeply through your left nostril during a rhythmic count of 4.

218. Keep your right nostril closed and now press your left one so that both are closed. Retain the air for a rhythmic count of 16.

219. Release your right nostril (your left one remains closed) and exhale slowly, deeply, and quietly during a rhythmic count of 8.

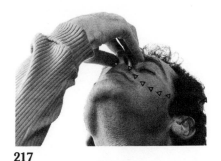

217

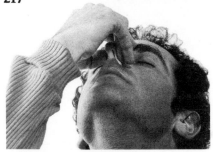

218

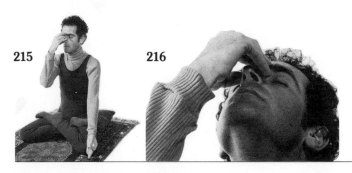

215   216

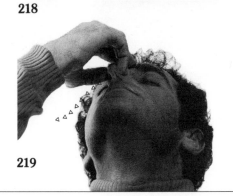

219

220. When the air is completely exhaled, press your right nostril so that both are closed, and *suspend breathing.* No air should enter during a rhythmic count of 4.

221. Release your right nostril and inhale a deep, quiet breath through your right nostril during a rhythmic count of 4.

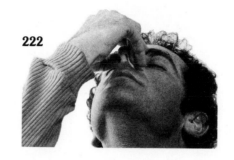

222. Keep your left nostril closed and now press your right one so that both are closed. Retain the air deep in your lungs during a rhythmic count of 16.

223. Release your left nostril (your right one remains closed) and exhale slowly, deeply, and quietly during a rhythmic count of 8.

224. Keep your right nostril closed and press your left one so that both are closed. *Suspend breathing.* No air should enter during a rhythmic count of 4.

This completes 1 round.

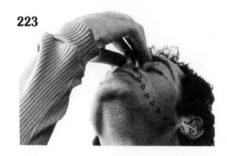

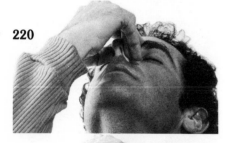

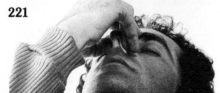

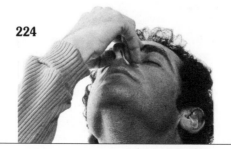

29th day

Without pause, keep your right nostril closed and begin the next round with a deep, quiet inhalation through your left nostril during a rhythmic count of 4.

Perform 7 rounds.

Lower your right hand and place it (in the *mudra*) on your right knee (or thigh). (Fig. 225.)

Summary

inhale through left	count 4
retain; both closed	count 16
exhale through right	count 8
suspend; both closed	count 4
without pause	
inhale through right	count 4
retain; both closed	count 16
exhale through left	count 8
suspend	count 4

This completes 1 round. Without pause, begin the next round.

Do not permit your breath to gush or hiss in or out. Perform the inhalations and exhalations as quietly as possible. Think of the breathing as occurring more in the throat than the nostrils.

The counting is rhythmic and continuous; it is never interrupted. Once the counting begins, you keep it going like a metronome, steady and rhythmic.

Throughout the exercise, your attention must be fully focused on the counting. It must not become automatic while your attention is allowed to wander. Total concentration on the counting, in conjunction with respiration, is the seed for this meditation practice.

When you have completed the 7 rounds, remain seated quietly for as long as you wish. You will note that your breathing is slow, your emotions quiet, your mind steady and one-pointed. It is in the state that one can begin to recognize what is meant in Yoga by *sat-chit-ananda*: existence-knowledge-bliss (Fig. 225.)

Open your eyes and extend your legs.

This terminates the meditation practice for today. (Make your notes.)

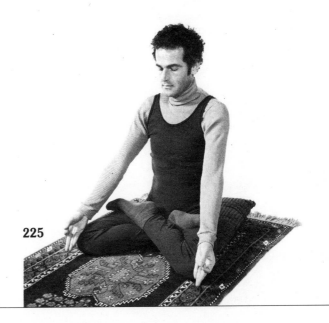

225

30th day
OM
(Mantra-Yantra)

The concluding technique of our *30 Day Plan* is the potent OM mantra-yantra combination. The individual values of each have been outlined previously. Now, in combining the two, there is a great energy generated that acts to elevate the consciousness not only during meditation, but for a considerable period of time thereafter. This fact is usually experienced by the student from his very first practice session with the OM mantra-yantra technique.

Both the external and internal vision are used for the yantra, and these are combined with both the audible and silent intonation of the mantra. The effectiveness of the technique will continue to increase as you develop ability in steady, one-pointed visualization, and as proficiency in breath and voice control enable you to intone the mantra with sufficient power.

Because of the manner in which inner awareness is heightened through the OM mantra-yantra, this technique is considered by many advanced students to be the ultimate meditation "with seed."

Perform Hatha Yoga Advanced Routine C page 167

Remain in the cross-legged posture. Open your eyes.

Place the book in a position where you may comfortably fix your gaze on Fig. 227. This was also the seed for the 25th Day.

Hold your gaze steadily on the figure for 5 minutes. Simultaneously, perform *audible* intonations of OM, as learned on the 20th Day. (Fig. 226.) The rhythm of the mantra remains at 4, 4-4-8, 2.

During each slow, complete inhalation, continue to gaze at the figure. Your attention can alternate between the figure and the sound. Eventually, these will merge, and your attention will be focused on that point of mergence.

When 5 minutes have elapsed, close your eyes and visualize the OM symbol. Simultaneously, without interrupting the rhythm you have established for the audible intonations, continue with *silent* repetitions of OM as practiced on the 20th Day. Your inner ear should hear the identical sound of OM as you performed it audibly. The rhythm remains the same. Your attention can alternate between the figure and the sound. Eventually, these will merge, and your attention will be focused on that point of mergence.

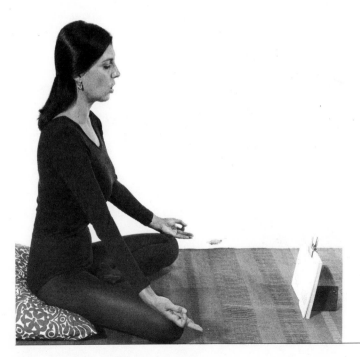

226. The audible-external practice. The gaze is fixed on the OM symbol while the OM mantra is *audibly* intoned.

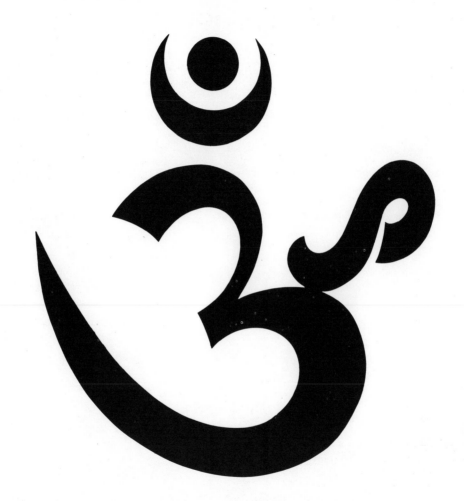

227. The symbol of OM.

30th day

Obviously, this technique requires intense concentration. If you lose either the image or the sound, pause for a moment, begin another inhalation, manifest the figure, and continue the practice. This internal-silent segment of the mantra-yantra technique is also practiced for 5 minutes. (Fig. 228.)

When the 5 minutes have elapsed, open your eyes and slowly extend your legs.

This terminates the meditation practice for today. (Make your notes.)

Important: Read the next page upon completion of your notes.

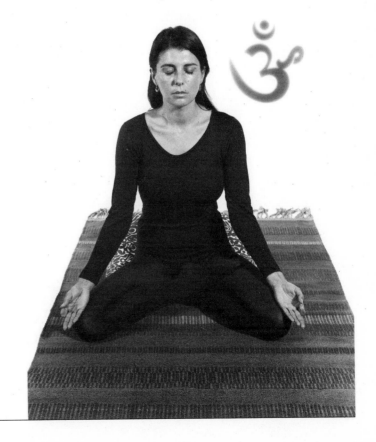

228. The silent-internal practice. The OM symbol is visualized while the mantra is *silently* intoned.

During the past 30 days, you have embarked upon a journey of the utmost significance. There has probably been sufficient light, here and there along the way, for you to glimpse some of the geography and recognize that there is no endeavor in this life that is more meaningful, or of greater value, than that which quiets the mind and turns it to traverse the path *inward*.

If you have indeed perceived the magnitude of this endeavor, you will also understand the necessity of continuing it *without interruption*. This means that having completed a segment of the journey today, you will begin another segment *tomorrow*. The form that this next segment should take will be determined by your reading the following pages prior to tomorrow's practice session. But regardless of the form, the message is clear: *daily practice is what is called for*. Nothing can be more urgent or more rewarding.

Continuing
Meditation

(1) The Selection of Three Techniques

Consulting your notes and your memory, you must now select the *three* meditation techniques that you have found to be the most meaningful and effective. The reason for utilizing three techniques at this point is to permit a more intensive concentration of energies (because of the reduced number) while still providing diversity in practice. This diversity alllows you to continue to experience the nuances of several forms of meditation. However, there are certain techniques that you have practiced during the 30 Day course, which, for reasons given in the next section, are not suited for Continuing Meditation and cannot be included in your selection of the three. Therefore, you must read this section and then refer to the second section, A Summary of the Techniques, before making your decisions.

Although there are students who, after the initial 30 days, can make their choices with certainty, the majority usually feels that additional sessions with almost all of the techniques are required in order to better determine the effects of these techniques. If the latter applies to your own situation, *you should not hesitate to repeat the course in its entirety, following all instructions exactly as presented, from the 1st to the 30th Day.* Even though there are techniques that cannot be included in your final selection of the three, they serve in several capacities and are to be practiced as part of the 30 Day course. If, at the conclusion of the second 30 days you are still uncertain, you can continue to repeat the course in its

entirety until three techniques suited for Continuing Meditation have clearly emerged.

In repeating the course, even several times, you do not in any way impede or delay what you may think of as progress. Actually, in the repetitions, you are continuing to meditate, continuing to learn the dynamics of steadying and quieting your mind while simultaneously determining which three techniques are, for you, the most meaningful. There is no advantage in proceeding with the practice plan of this section, which utilizes the three techniques, until you are certain that you have those three which merit your total commitment in terms of serious, regular practice on an extended basis. Such a commitment is essential for one's continuing to benefit from meditation.

Therefore, you must now decide whether or not you can choose three techniques with the certainty that has been indicated above. If you *cannot* do so, begin at the 1st Day (following the 30th Day *without interruption*) and, in the next 30 days, repeat the course in its entirety. In each *asana* of the Hatha Yoga Routines, perform the most advanced position of which you are now capable. Also, at the conclusion of each day's meditation practice, continue to make your notes. (In many of the techniques, your new notes may differ from those you made previously. You have undergone certain changes during the course of your practice, therefore your experiences with the various techniques may be correspond-

ingly altered. Your notes can always be an important factor when you are considering your selection of the techniques for Continuing Meditation, so as often as you repeat the course, keep a record of your experiences. This should be done at the conclusion of each session, even though the technique of that day may not be one that is suited for Continuing Meditation.) If, as of today, you *are able* to make your selection of the three techniques, then refer to the next section, A Summary of the Techniques, to determine whether all three are suited for Continuing Meditation. If any (or all) are not, substitute as necessary. If you cannot make this substitution with the same certainty you had in your original selection(s), do not hesitate to repeat the course until the required number of techniques emerge.

In the next section, you will find the method to be employed for Continuing Meditation with each technique that is suited for such practice. Having made your final selection of the three techniques (now, or 30, 60, 90, 120, etc. days hence), refer to the appropriate pages in the next section—those which contain the instructions for Continuing Meditation with the techniques you have chosen—and proceed accordingly.

Let's assume that you have gone through the 30 Day course twice, and although you have continued to develop ability in the overall technique of meditating, and you have derived the benefits inherent in learning how to quiet your mind and turn it inward, you are still unable to make a definite selection of three techniques. Perhaps one or two have prominently emerged but not three. Therefore, you repeat the course again. Upon your third completion, you clearly established that Candle (2), OM (3), and Yantra (5)* are the three techniques that have proven most meaningful and

*These are totally arbitrary selections by the author for the purpose of presenting an example of the practice plan and should in no way influence the reader's selections.

effective. (The terms "meaningful" and "effective," are used here only to indicate several possible effects of the techniques that might influence your selection. However, you may not wish to think about your meditation experiences in any descriptive terms whatsoever. If this is the case, you simply determine to which of the three techniques you find yourself intuitively drawn. Such attraction, if it is definite, is certainly sufficient basis upon which to make your selection. Your intuition is always to be trusted.) You would then incorporate these three techniques, together with the *asana* routines, into a rotating plan for Continuing Meditation.

Here is an example of such a plan:

Day	Asana Routine	Meditation
June 1	A	Candle (2)
June 2	B	OM (3)
June 3	C	Yantra (5)
June 4	A	Candle (2)
June 5	B	OM (3)
June 6	C	Yantra (5)
June 7	A	Candle (2)
etc.	etc.	etc.
Sept. 1		On this date (three months from the time you began the above practice plan) you must refer to the third section on page 215 and continue your meditation accordingly.

Referring to the above example, make a chart that includes the proper dates and techniques, so that on any given day, you will know your exact plan of practice. Include the date on which the three months of practice will be concluded (at which time you will undertake the practice plan presented in the third section).

> The following information pertains to Continuing Meditation with both the above plan (utilizing three techniques) and the Primary plan that is the subject of the third section. Certain information that has previously appeared in the text is also included here in the interest of clarity, so that the student will have no doubts as to how to proceed. This information should be carefully studied.

It may be that you can execute the advanced positions of some *asanas* but only the elementary or intermediate positions of others. Continue to work toward the advanced positions in all of the *asanas*, including the attainment of the Half and Full Lotus, and the ability to remain in these, without discomfort, during the entire meditation period.

If you have been using a Hatha Yoga practice plan from one of my other books, you may continue to do so. Any Hatha Yoga routine that has proven effective for you is satisfactory. Now simply add the appropriate meditation technique to the end of the routine(s). But remember that Observation of the Breath must always immediately precede meditation.

If you are meditating twice daily, you need to perform the *asana* routine in one session only (it can be either session). The *asana* routine in the other session is optional. If you are performing an *asana* routine that is longer than those in this book, you may divide that routine between the two sessions. But remember that Observation of the Breath must precede meditation in both sessions.

From time to time, you may question your choice of techniques: you wonder if it is still a valid choice, and you find yourself considering the efficacy of changing techniques. At such times, remember that your selection was made following a significant period of practice and learning. Therefore, you can remain confident that this choice is the correct one. Actually, at this more advanced point in your practice, you derive little from the technique(s); it now serves as the vehicle for continued development and refinement of perception, awareness, consciousness. If doubts as to the validity of the technique arise, it is because you think you are not making satisfactory progress, or that certain anticipated results have not manifested. But the serious meditator does not look for results from his meditation practice. To the beginner, this statement may seem peculiar because results are sought in any and all worldly activities. People act in particular ways, hoping that these actions will produce the anticipated results. But our objectives in meditation are altogether different from those which we seek to attain, through action, in daily life. Meditation produces what may be described as a metamorphosis, a transformation through *inaction*. Understanding this, the meditator is not troubled with the anticipation of results. He knows that what is required is not the changing of techniques, but his continued patient, serious, and regular practice with the technique(s) originally chosen.

You must not attempt to judge or evaluate your progress in the practice of meditation. Degrees of achievement *can* be noted with respect to the *asanas:* because you are continually aware of the condition of your body, your accomplishments in the postures are obvious. It is a simple matter to judge how far you have advanced and how far you may still have to go to achieve the more advanced positions. But in meditation, the concept of progress, like that of action, has no application. You *will* gradually become aware of *transformation,* what is designated by certain teachers as "an expansion of consciousness," and you will recognize the absolute impossibility of describing this condition or relating it to the ordinary person's definitions of results and progress. The element of time is equally nonapplicable. Although it appears that all we do, including our Yoga and meditation practice, is transpiring within periods of time, and although the instructions in this

book specify various time segments, as the depth of perception increases, the meditator understands that time is a concept of the ordinary mind and that he, in union with the Eternal (Yoga), does not exist in time. I make this point here to impress upon the student that because progress and results are illusions of the ordinary mind, the amount of time he believes he is devoting to meditation is totally inconsequential. The serious student gives no consideration to the number of days, months, or years he has been involved in meditation. It is the *practice,* not the illusion of progress, that becomes his primary concern.

It must now be obvious that daily practice is imperative. Everyone knows the regularity of practice and dedication that are necessary for developing the necessary skills to become proficient in almost any field. How much more so is it in gaining the ability to quiet the mind and turn it inward. Daily practice, preferably shortly after rising and, again, later in the day, should become a well-established pattern. During the initial months of practice, your ordinary mind will present every possible excuse—from the most subtle to the most obvious—to prevent you from undertaking regular, daily practice. The ordinary mind recognizes the great threat to its position of dominance that is inherent in this practice and will utilize all of its resources in diverting you from it. As the hour for practice approaches, the most insignificant activity that may delay or cancel the session suddenly assumes the greatest urgency in your ordinary mind. But if you can overcome these contrivances and persevere in your practice at the scheduled hour for approximately six months, you will no longer be subject to the ordinary mind's diversions in this area because at that point the situation is reversed: *nothing is of greater importance than your meditation practice.*

In addition to the ordinary mind's diversionary tactics described in the previous paragraph, there will be days on which, during the actual meditation session, it seems especially difficult to control the mind and bring it to focus in the desired one-pointed manner. Like a wild stallion which, when it realizes it is being contained, will race frantically in all directions to escape, so will the ordinary mind, when it periodically "gets the message" that you are serious about restraining its wild ramblings, wage a particularly strong rebellion against such restraint. This situation is universal among beginning meditators, and it is extremely important that you recognize such periods—which can have a duration of from one to several consecutive sessions—not as regressions in achieving your one-pointed objective, but as an almost inevitable aspect of the "taming the mind" process. Simply continue your practice with patience during these more trying times; they soon pass, and you will find that your mind is then more receptive to control than it was prior to the period of turmoil! I emphasize this point so that you will never become discouraged when you are experiencing what the ordinary mind—the very entity that is creating the turmoil—will attempt to interpret as a setback or a lack of progress.

Circumstances may arise (illness, travel, and so forth) in which you are unable to or do not wish to assume the cross-legged position and practice in your accustomed manner. In these situations, you can usually accommodate your practice in bed by closing your eyes and performing the pertinent technique silently, to the best of your ability. If you are utilizing flower, incense, touch, candle, or certain other seeds for meditation, it may be necessary to eliminate these temporarily and substitute Observation of the Breath, internal visualization, or the silent OM. Through substitutions or minor adjustments, you should be able to meditate under almost any circumstances.

If, on occasion, you are deeply absorbed in meditation, and you sense that it is necessary to terminate this condition, simply open your eyes and perform several deep (complete) breaths. Avoid the abrupt termination of a meditation session. If you are ever startled by anything that occurs during meditation, do not become alarmed. You can either terminate

the session by opening your eyes and performing the breathing, or you can turn such an occurrence to your advantage by asking "Who is experiencing this phenomenon?" With this question, you immediately divert the focus of attention from the phenomenon; you drive the mind inward to investigate the nature of the ego and discover the illusion of the "I." If there is no "I," who is it that can be startled or alarmed? When the interruption has passed, resume your practice.

Is there a particular way of life conducive to meditation, that facilitates attainment of its objectives? In other books, I have treated life-style, conduct, morality, and the like as they pertain to the everyday life of the Yoga student, and I have always stressed that these things cannot be structured according to preconceived notions of what constitutes the correct and incorrect paths, but must emerge, in a totally natural manner, as the result of having reestablished contact with Self. In this contact, the direction that all aspects of his life

should take is clearly perceived by the meditator; he soon comes to Know that his questions are answered, and his problems resolved, during the course of patient meditation. There is no guidance as certain as that which comes when the mind is quieted and turned inward.

Again, I advise that you do not discuss your meditation practice with anyone. Such discussion is of no value and only dissipates vital energies. The transformation of consciousness occurs in the deepest silence, and one must not intrude upon it. Whatever further guidance you may require for fruitful practice will be forthcoming from this silence.

With the beginning student, we use the expression "practicing meditation." But the more advanced student recognizes meditation as his natural and *sole* state of existence. The beginner distinguishes between his regular activities and that time when he meditates; the accomplished meditator can make no such distinction for he knows that whatever he does proceeds only from the meditative state.

(2) A Summary of the Techniques

This section describes those techniques which are suited for Continuing Meditation and those which are to be utilized in other contexts. Carefully study this summary before making your final selection of the three techniques.

Deep Relaxation (1st, 15th, & 22nd days)

The Feeling of Deep Relaxation (1st day)

This technique is meant to serve as *preparation* for meditation rather than for the practice of meditation on an extended basis. It is of great value in relieving physical, emotional, and mental tensions and anxieties. Whenever

necessary, it can be used for these purposes as well as for helping to induce a restful sleep, for dealing with pain and depression, and in preparing for a demanding business, scholastic, social, or sports event.

As indicated on the 1st Day, once having experienced deep relaxation, and recognizing the point from which the *feeling* of the relaxation is emanating, this point can be contacted with increasing ease and frequency. You may already be able to make such contact simply by sitting or lying quietly for a few moments, withdrawing your senses, and remembering the feeling of the deeply relaxed state. The instant the contact is made, you find yourself relaxed. Eventually, the relaxed state can become your *natural* state; its immediacy and depth increase with practice. Therefore, while it is not to be included in your selection of techniques for Continuing Meditation, you can utilize Deep Relaxation whenever necessary for the purposes indicated above, and also continue to develop your aptitude in its application by periodically including it in your Hatha Yoga routines.

When included in the *asana* routines, the technique is to be performed exactly as instructed on the 1st Day; the "feeling" segment remains at 5 minutes. But when applying it for therapy (relief of tension, for example), or for a specific purpose during the course of daily activities (prior to an important meeting, examination, tennis game), any physical position (sitting or even standing) is acceptable, and the "feeling" segment may be shortened or lengthened according to the circumstances. With a little practice, you will learn how to make the contact in almost any physical position and, if conditions dictate, with your eyes open.

Deep Relaxation: a Path to the Void (15th day)

This technique is suited for Continuing Meditation. It is to be utilized exactly as instructed on the 15th Day. The 5-minute "void" segment may be lengthened as desired. Both the objectives and instructions should be read regularly.

Visualization of Perfect Health During Deep Relaxation (22nd day)

As with The Feeling of Deep Relaxation, this technique is utilized primarily for therapeutic purposes. It can be highly effective in the maintenance and restoration of health and should be applied in this context as necessary. It it not suited for Continuing Meditation.

Candle (2nd & 19th days)

The Candle technique of the 2nd Day is preparatory for the more advanced work. In Continuing Meditation, only the technique of the 19th Day is utilized. Practice it exactly as instructed there. Both the objectives and instructions should be read regularly.

White Light (3rd & 24th days)

Of the two White Light techniques, that of the 3rd Day is suited for Continuing Meditation. Although on the 3rd Day we have designated the technique as effective for "revitalizing," when it is used on a continuing basis, your attention is fully focused on the visualization of the white light and no thought need be given to the revitalization effects. These effects are automatic. Therefore, simply eliminate the revitalization concept and practice exactly as instructed on the 3rd Day.

The technique of the 24th Day is to be applied in healing and recovery situations. When utilized for these purposes, the white light must be visualized flowing into the afflicted area.

Yantras (4th, 8th, 12th, 16th, 21st, & 25th days)

Any of the yantras can be used for Continuing Meditation.

In selecting a yantra, practice to gradually achieve the following objectives:

1. During the first segment of the daily session (fixing the gaze on the yantra), see the figure *in its entirety*. Dispense with the observation of the individual configurations—lines, circles, dots—and absorb the *total* yantra during the entire period (2 minutes or 5 minutes) allotted for the external practice. (This technique was instructed on the 21st and 25th Days.)

2. With continued visualization practice, the impression of the yantra eventually becomes so firmly established in the consciousness that the assistance of the external image is no longer required and can be eliminated as the first part of the session. You can then begin the meditation simply by closing your eyes and manifesting the total yantra. The entire meditation session, of whatever length you wish, is devoted solely to this practice.

(Both of the above objectives are achieved *gradually*. As you work toward these objectives, continue to utilize any expedient that has been provided in the various yantra Instructions for assisting you in the development and strengthening of visualization.)

Yantra meditation requires intensive concentration, and in longer sessions, the practice should be terminated when

you begin to experience fatigue, not restlessness or distraction. There is a fine line here, and you will learn to distinguish between them. You will find that your ability in sustaining this concentration varies from day to day; this is natural, and you must never be discouraged if your visualization is weak on a particular day. Simply practice to the best of your ability on that day and recognize that an occasional weak session is a natural link in the growth process.

There comes a time when the effort required for manifestation of the yantra is minimal. As you close your eyes, it is already there, or will appear almost instantly. At this point, you can allow the yantra to be and do as it will. It may manifest in color, it may be large or small, it may move or vibrate. Simply observe whatever is occurring. If it invites you to merge with it, do so. The general significance and value of yantra meditation are first outlined on the 4th Day, and you should read that section regularly as well as the objectives and instructions of the particular yantra you have selected for meditation.

Yantras are also suited for meditation at any time of the day you find yourself in a "waiting" situation, or when you need a brief period of relaxation. Regardless of where you are, simply close your eyes and practice your visualization. The yantra you have chosen will gradually become a source of energy and illumination, and you will look forward to contact with it.

Alternate Nostril Breathing (5th, 11th, 18th, & 29th days)

The final form of this technique, as instructed on the 29th Day, is the one for Continuing Meditation practice. However, you may select Alternate Nostril Breathing for Continuing Meditation even if you have not yet perfected the technique in its final form. In this case, you will work successively with its three preceding forms (5th, 11th, and 18th Days) to gain the necessary proficiency for the ultimate practice.

(Note that Alternate Nostril Breathing is utilized by those who are serious students of Laya-Kundalini Yoga as one of the techniques for uniting the *prana* and *apana* currents [*vayus*] and directing them into the *sushumna* canal. Although this is not an objective in our practice of Alternate Nostril Breathing, the reader who is interested in *kundalini* should refer to my book *Yoga: The 8 Steps to Health and Peace.* *)

The objectives of Alternate Nostril Breathing that concern us in this 30 Day course appear in the text of the days indicated above. These as well as the instructions for the practice of the form with which you are working should be read regularly.

*Hittleman, *loc. cit.*

OM (6th, 13th, & 20th days)

The completed technique, as instructed on the 20th Day, is the one for Continuing Meditation practice. Both the audible and silent segments are practiced in each session, and both may be lengthened to as many repetitions (*japa*) as you

wish. The "quiet observation" period following the practice may also be lengthened.

The internal intonation is suited for meditation at any time of the day that you find yourself in a "waiting" situation, or when you need a brief period of relaxation. Simply close your eyes and silently intone the OM mantra.

The instructions of the 20th Day as well as the general information in the texts of the 6th, 13th, and 20th Days should be read regularly.

OM (Mantra-Yantra) (30th day)

Continue with this technique exactly as instructed on the 30th Day.

Both the audible-external and silent-internal segments are to be included in each practice session. The latter is also suited for meditation in those situations described on the 20th Day.

The objectives and instructions should be read regularly.

Asana Meditation (7th, 14th, & 27th days)

As you continue to practice the *asanas,* their movements become increasingly easy. When you are no longer involved with learning the movements, your attention is freed to be focused in a way that will not only increase the *effectiveness* of the *asanas,* but serve as a highly meaningful form of meditation. You have already applied this technique of Asana Meditation on the 7th, 14th, and 27th Days. We now recommend that as soon as you feel comfortable with the routines, you apply this technique to each *asana.* In this way, *your entire Hatha Yoga practice becomes meditative.* All of the pertinent information appears in the text of the 7th Day, and this should be read regularly.

Asana Meditation is not to be selected for Continuing Meditation. It is applied in your Hatha Yoga routines to provide the benefits of additional meditation as well as to increase the effectiveness of the *asanas.*

(Those students who are following the practice plan of my book *Yoga: The 8 Steps To Health And Peace**—which includes the visualization of the yantras during *asana* practice—can continue to do so. The "primary" meditation technique that you will ultimately select from this 30 Day course is simply added to the end of those routines. Remember, however, that Observation of the Breath must always precede meditation.)

*Hittleman, *loc. cit.*

Active Meditation (9th & 23rd days)

The movements—and visualizations—of the Complete Breath Standing *asana* are meant to serve as the *experience* of a cyclic progression. The value of this is explained in the texts of the 9th and 23rd Days. Active Meditation is not suited

for Continuing Meditation, but it is a valuable technique to now include in your Hatha Yoga practice. If your time permits, it should be included as an *asana* in one or in all three of the daily routines. So that you will not forget this technique, write "Active Meditation: The Complete Breath Standing" at that point in the routine(s) where it will be performed. This is left to the student's discretion. Remember that there are two different visualizations (9th and 23rd Days), and you may select either of them or alternate both. As one of the *asanas* of a routine, only the first segment of Active Meditation need be performed. Of course, if your time permits, the passive segment may also be included.

Read the objectives and instructions for visualization regularly.

Meditation With the Senses (10th, 17th, & 26th days)

The Flower, Incense, and Touch techniques are suited for Continuing Meditation.

Flower (10th day)

Practice exactly as instructed on the 10th Day. Although it is ideal to use the same kind of flower for each session, from time to time you may have to make a change (due to season, availability, and so forth). In this event, any flower that is pleasing to you will be satisfactory. You should then attempt to use *that* variety of flower for as long as circumstances permit. The flower that is used for the meditation session can either remain in the practice area or be placed where your eyes will fall upon it occasionally during the day.

Both the objectives and instructions should be read regularly.

Incense (17th day)

Practice exactly as instructed on the 17th Day. Although it is ideal to use the same scent and brand of incense for each session, it is possible that circumstances (availability) may make a change necessary. In this event, any incense that you find pleasing will be satisfactory. When making your pur- chase, obtain as large a quantity as is practical. The meditation incense generally can be used in your environment at other times of the day.

Both the objectives and instructions should be read regularly.

Touch (26th day)

Practice exactly as instructed on the 26th Day. The object that you have originally chosen should be used for each session. Following practice, it should be covered or placed in a container. No one else should be permitted to contact this object. In the event it is misplaced or lost, select as similar an object as possible.

The text of the 26th Day should be read regularly.

Hansa-Soham: The Involuntary Mantras (28th day)

In Continuing Meditation, this technique is applied to Observation of the Breath that previously has preceded each meditation session. Now with the application of *hansa-soham*, Observation of the Breath *becomes* the meditation and can be utilized as the concluding technique of each daily Hatha Yoga routine. It is to be practiced exactly as instructed on the 28th Day.

Observation of the Breath is also suited for practice at any time of the day you wish to quiet your mind. Regardless of where you are, direct your attention to your breathing and hear the mantras *hansa-soham*.

For Continuing Meditation

Deep Relaxation: A Path to the Void—15th Day (See also page 208.)

Candle (2)—19th Day (See also page 208.)

White Light (1)—3rd Day (See also page 209.)

Flower—10th Day (See also page 212.)

Incense—17th Day (See also page 212.)

Touch—26th Day (See also page 212.)

Alternate Nostril Breathing (4)—29th Day (See also page 210.)

Yantras (All) (See also page 209.)

OM (3)—20th Day (See also page 210.)

OM Mantra-Yantra—30th Day (See also page 210.)

Hansa-Soham: The Involuntary Mantras—28th Day (See also page 212.)

For Use as Needed

The Feeling of Deep Relaxation—1st Day (See also page 207.)

Visualization of Perfect Health During Deep Relaxation—22nd Day (See also page 208.)

White Light (2)—24th Day (See also page 209.)

Miscellaneous

Active Meditation—9th & 23rd Days: To be included in any one or more of the *asana* routines (See also page 211.)

Asana Meditation—7th, 14th, & 27th Days: To be applied in all Hatha Yoga practice (See also page 211.)

(3) Selection of the Primary Technique

Having concluded three months of practice with the plan utilizing three techniques, you are in a position to further refine your selection. From the three techniques, now select the *one* that has emerged as most effective, most meaningful, or that simply holds the strongest attraction. This *one* becomes your primary technique, and you work with it exclusively from this point on. It serves as the vehicle through which the ultimate objective of meditation is achieved.

Let's assume that of the three techniques you previously selected and have been utilizing in your practice during the past three months, OM (3) is your choice for the primary technique.* You incorporate this technique into a Continuing Meditation plan that must include the daily rotation of the *asana* routines.

*An arbitrary selection by the author, which should not influence the reader's selection.

Day	Asana Routine	Meditation
Sept. 1	A	OM
Sept. 2	B	OM
Sept. 3	C	OM
Sept. 4	A	OM
etc.	etc.	etc.

The information on pages 204–207 pertains equally to this Primary Technique plan and should be read regularly. Whatever additional guidance may be necessary will be forthcoming in the course of your patient, regular meditation practice. Those who meditate seriously always receive the guidance they require. Of this, you need never have the slightest doubt.

About the Author

Richard Hittleman is the world's most widely read author on the subject of Yoga. Following many years of intensive study and practice of Oriental disciplines, he began his instruction of Yoga in the early 1950s. He has written twelve books on the various aspects of Yoga, and his *Yoga for Health* television programs are seen throughout the United States and in many foreign countries.

Mr. Hittleman conducts intensive Yoga Workshops several times each year in the vicinity of his northern California residence. He is currently preparing a new television series in which he will instruct the techniques of meditation.

Readers who are interested in receiving information regarding Mr. Hittleman's meditation record album may write to:

Yoga for Health, P. O. Box 475, Carmel, California 93921

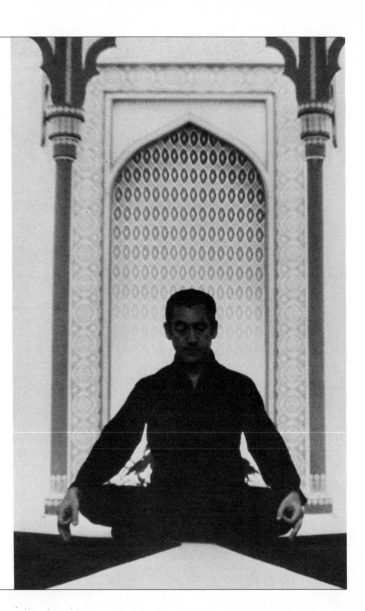